50 Questions
(You MUST Ask!)
Before You Have
Plastic Surgery

Who is the
aenesthicologrst

Brenton B. Koch, MD, FACS

Southfork Publishing
Brenton Koch, MD, FACS
4855 Mills Civic Parkway, Suite 100
West Des Moines, IA 50265
(515) 277-5555
Koch@kochmd.com

Printed in the United States of America

First Printing, 2012

ISBN-13: 978-1480236660

ISBN-10: 1480236667

Cover design by Sumit Shringi

The information contained in this book is intended to provide helpful and informative material on the subject addressed. It is not intended to serve as a replacement for professional medical advice. Any use of the information in this book is at the reader's discretion. The author and publisher specifically disclaim any and all liability arising directly or indirectly from the use or application of any information contained in this book. A health care professional should be consulted regarding your specific situation. Bottom line; ask your doctor.

Table of Contents

This book is dedicated to the people who have given me the ability to write it – my patients. My patients inspire me, challenge me, puzzle me, and make me laugh. But most importantly, they teach me. My patients teach me that caring for someone else is not a task – it is an honor.

Dwell on the beauty of life. Watch the stars, and see yourself running with them.

Marcus Aurelias

Introduction

Beauty surrounds us.

Rumi

This is an exciting time for everyone in the cosmetic surgery field. Technology in medicine and surgery is leaps and bounds ahead of where it was when I started my facial plastic and reconstructive surgery practice fourteen years ago, and a steady parade of new products and less invasive procedures has made it possible for more people than ever to attain the face and body of their dreams. According to the American Society of Plastic Surgeons, the number of cosmetic procedures in the United States has doubled since the year 2000. In 2011 alone, there were nearly fourteen million cosmetic procedures done in America.[1] So if you are walking down the street in a major metroplex thinking that you're the only one considering plastic surgery, you couldn't

---

[1] www.plasticsurgery.org/Documents/news-resources/statistics/2011-statistics/2011_Stats_Quick_Facts.pdf, accessed September 26, 2012.

be more wrong. You probably just walked past five other folks who were thinking about exactly the same thing. That's the new reality. There is a huge demand for cosmetic procedures, and consumers are spending billions of dollars on them each year.

When demand for a product or service increases, we all know what happens: the supply side does whatever it has to do to keep pace, and opportunists come up with all kinds of creative ways to wrangle a piece of the pie for themselves. The multi-billion dollar plastic surgery industry is no exception. Laser shops have suddenly started springing up in strip malls from coast to coast. Doctors with little or no training in plastic surgery are now offering surgical and nonsurgical cosmetic procedures in hopes of making a quick buck. Cosmetic procedures have become a consumer-driven, commoditized big business.

The increasing popularity of cosmetic procedures brings both good and bad news for you as a potential patient. The good news: *there is a ton of information out there to help you become a better informed consumer*. The bad news? *There is a ton of information out there designed to confuse and deceive you.*

If you have been even the slightest bit interested in having plastic surgery for any length of time, you have probably encountered a mountain of both kinds of information already. You may have read about other people's experiences with plastic surgery on the Internet, in books, in magazines and in the newspaper – and it's likely that almost all of those were horror stories, because patients who are happy with their outcomes rarely alert the media. Think about it. Have you ever seen anyone on YouTube say, "Look at me! I'm perfectly normal!"? Perhaps you have watched news accounts and listened to radio programs discussing the latest industry trends. You've probably learned about (pardon the pun) cutting-edge procedures and treatments in brochures, flyers, prime time television commercials and late night infomercials. You may have watched reality shows, YouTube videos and documentaries that took you straight into the operating room to witness actual cosmetic surgeries in all their gory glory.

But here's the thing as you contemplate having your own plastic surgery: how does any of that information apply to you as an individual? How do you even begin to distinguish fact from fiction? How do you decide which procedure is the right one for you? How can you know which doctor and facility are the best choices for your chosen procedure? How can you increase the odds of getting the results you want? How can you be sure you are even a good candidate for plastic surgery in the first place?

Every day, patients come to me with all kinds of preconceived notions based upon completely false information about plastic surgery. And every day, patients come to me for consultations and have absolutely no questions for me at all. They say, "You tell me what I need, and let's get it done." Whenever that happens, I am stunned that that is the extent of the information they are seeking. I am astonished that they are ready to write a five-digit check and let someone they just met alter their appearance forever, without asking any questions whatsoever. It blows me off my chair every time it happens.

Patients often come to me for help after bad procedures with other doctors and they say things like, "Is this result normal?" and "I didn't realize that my nose would look like THIS afterward!" or "I had no idea that my doctor had only done one or two of these surgeries a year." I don't hear this kind of thing just once in a blue moon, mind you. I hear it at least once a month, and the number of disappointed patients seems to be increasing exponentially lately.

But there is a flip side of those unfortunate scenarios, and that is the patient who comes into the consultation carrying a legal pad filled from front to back with questions they want answered. As long as an attorney does not accompany that legal pad, and as long as those questions are within reason, I know right then and there that they are going to be an excellent patient. They are going to end up pleased with their results. The more factual information the patient collects, the better off the patient, the surgeon, the anesthesiologist and the support staff are going to be. More factual information is good; inaccurate or little information is downright scary.

You are a human being, not a dollar sign. You are someone's wife, mother, brother, son, sister, grandmother, friend. You owe it to yourself and to your loved ones to get all the facts straight before you undergo any procedure, no matter how simple it may seem. If I seem preachy right now, it's because I feel so strongly about this. I am not exaggerating when I say that getting the right information up front can literally save your life. If you make an uninformed decision about your procedure with someone who does things in an unsafe fashion in an unsafe facility without proper support, it can be a decision that you and everyone who loves you will regret forever.

That is the outcome I am trying to prevent with this book.

In the pages that follow, I am going to cut through all the fluff and confusion and tell you in straightforward, honest terms exactly what to ask potential surgeons and their support staff during your plastic surgery consultation. Together, you and I will walk through a list of questions that has been fourteen years in the making; a series of inquiries designed to bring you greater clarity and confidence as a potential consumer of plastic surgery. These are the questions I get on a day-to-day basis from those well-prepared patients I described above. These are the questions I wish all of my patients would ask me. And not only am I going to give you the questions, but I am also going to give you the answers that I think are the most responsible and helpful. Lastly, I am going to give you a series of questions for you to ask **yourself** about your motivation, expectations and readiness for plastic surgery. These are the questions I wish all of my patients would ask themselves before they come in for a consultation.

My goal with this book is to neither talk you into nor out of having plastic surgery. My only goal is to provide you with the necessary tools for getting all the information you need for making sound choices. Do not be shy about asking these questions. Stand up for your right to know. Do not allow any doctor or staff member to make you feel like you're being unreasonable because you're making these inquiries. Never forget that you are the customer in this plastic surgery "store." This store owes you terrific service and personalized details about the product they are trying to sell you. That's the bottom line.

Plastic surgery is serious business. This is not like coloring your hair. This is not like getting your house painted. You can re-paint your house and you can re-color your hair if you don't like the initial results, but plastic surgery is a one-way street. It is a point of no return. To do it safely, you must go into it with your eyes wide open and your brain fully engaged. You must go down that road with a detailed map to guide you. This book is your starting point on that all-important journey. I wish you safe and happy travels!

QUESTIONS TO ASK YOUR SURGEON

First things first…

Question 1: Why is it called "plastic" surgery?

Patients often ask me if I will be putting plastic into their face during their surgery. The answer is a resounding no! Here's the scoop on why the procedure is called plastic surgery:

When certain chemicals are mixed in a certain way, they create polymers that are moldable. The creators of some polymers decided to call them "plastics," which is a descriptive term derived from the Greek word *plasticos*, meaning "changeable" and "moldable."

Actual plastics (such as those used to create soda bottles, milk jugs and margarine tubs) have nothing to do with your surgery. Your procedure is called plastic surgery because it creates visible change. It is a procedure that reforms a body part – such as a nose or a breast – following a disease, or after a patient has made a cosmetic choice to do so. The surgeon molds some part of the body into a different form, and that is the basis for the term "plastic" surgery.

Therefore, you can rest assured that no margarine tubs will be harmed in the making of your new nose.

The Surgeon's Qualifications

Happy girls are the prettiest.

Audrey Hepburn

Question 2: What is your board certification?

You want to be certain that your surgeon is qualified to perform the procedure(s) you are seeking, so the first step is to ask about his/her board certification. To be board certified in a particular medical specialty means that the doctor has completed a certain amount of focused training, passed exams and participated in continuing education to maintain their certification.

For example, a surgeon might be board certified in general surgery and then later do a fellowship or training in plastic surgery, thereby becoming board certified in that as well. An ophthalmologist can obtain an additional board certification by doing a fellowship in oculoplastic surgery. A board-certified dermatologist might also become certified in cosmetic dermatology involving resurfacing the skin. In my case, I was initially board certified in ear, nose, and throat (ENT) surgery, and immediately thereafter I did a fellowship surgery. So I have dual board certification in

,d facial plastic surgery.

,ck to make sure that your surgeon's certifications
are current. Make certain that the certifications are from
reputable boards and not strange fly-by-night outfits. Do
some digging, especially if the board is **not** one of the
following, which are the most common, highly regarded
boards for plastic surgeons in the United States:

- American Board of Plastic Surgery (ABPS):
  www.abplsurg.org
- American Board of Cosmetic Surgery (ABCS):
  www.americanboardcosmeticsurgery.org
- American Board of Facial Plastic and
  Reconstructive Surgery (ABFPRS):
  www.abfprs.org
- American Board of Medical Specialties
  (ABMS): www.abms.org
- American Board of Dermatology:
  www.abderm.org
- American Board of Oral and Maxillofacial
  Surgery (ABOMS): www.aboms.org

Each of the above websites has a locator feature that
will help you find board-certified physicians in your area.

Question 3: Of which professional societies are you a member?

Each surgical specialty has societies that bestow various honors and membership degrees upon their members. Being a recognized member of a society is a signal that the surgeon has completed a certain level of education and training in his or her specialty. Here are some of the most common societies for plastic surgeons in the United States:

- American Society of Plastic Surgeons (ASPS®): www.plasticsurgery.org
- American Society for Aesthetic Plastic Surgery (ASAPS): www.surgery.org
- American Society of Ophthalmic Plastic and Reconstructive Surgery (ASOPRS): www.asoprs.org
- American College of Surgeons: www.facs.org
- Academy of Facial Plastic and Reconstructive Surgeons www.afprs.org

One final note on board certification and societies: a surgeon can be board certified and be a member of a prestigious society and still not be particularly great at the kind of surgery you are seeking. Checking certifications and memberships is only the first step in your investigation into a surgeon's qualifications. If the surgeon you are considering has shaky credentials, consider it a major red flag and cross him off your list. On the other hand, if a surgeon has great credentials, mark that as a plus and proceed with your inquiry.

Question 4: What is your recent experience performing the procedure you are recommending for me? How many of these procedures do you do each year?

Let's say you're about to board a Boeing 787 Dreamliner airplane for an overseas flight to Japan. Which scenario would make you feel more comfortable: knowing that your pilot has flown that same aircraft hundreds of times and flies it four or five times each week, or that she has only flown it once in her career? Surely you would feel better knowing that she has flown that plane every day for years. You'd feel more at ease knowing that your pilot is familiar with the controls; that she understands the tilts and the glide patterns and the quirks of that particular plane... and that she knows exactly what to do should a problem arise.

Surgery is no different. When a surgeon focuses on certain procedures and does them over and over again every day, she gains experience. That experience is golden. By practicing the same procedures repeatedly, the surgeon has the opportunity to perfect her approach and to learn from her mistakes – and believe me, we all make mistakes. Surgeons are people, too.

In his book OUTLIERS, author Malcolm Gladwell examined a fascinating concept called the 10,000-Hour Rule. Gladwell wrote that studies have shown that mastering any discipline, whether it is music, sports, or computer programming, for example, requires 10,000 hours of focused, deliberate practice. Once you reach that 10,000-hour point – usually at around five to seven years of intensive study and practice – the activity becomes almost second nature. And once the technical aspects of the activity are mastered, the practitioner's body and mind are free to get creative and express the *art* of whatever it is they do. I believe that the 10,000-Hour Rule applies to surgery, too. In my own case, I know that after fourteen years doing facial plastic surgery, I am technically stronger and more confident than I was when I first started.

Experience helps, but it isn't the only important factor. On the very first day that wide receiver Randy Moss walked out onto the football field as a rookie NFL player, he was the best wide receiver in the league. Moss didn't have any professional experience, but he had extraordinary talent. There were other guys in the league who had played the wide receiver position for years, yet they could never approach the proficiency of Randy Moss at that time.

There are inexperienced surgeons with extraordinary talent as well, but your odds of success are better if your surgeon has been practicing your procedure for some time.

If you ask your potential surgeon how much experience he has with your procedure and his response is that he learned it last month at a weekend seminar, I recommend that you head for the door. There is no reason to take a gamble with a rookie, unless you have seen the rookie's talent. That one rookie may be a "first round draft pick." Just do your research and make informed decisions.

Question 5: May I see recent before-and-after photographs of your past patients' results?

If a surgeon is not willing to show you some before-and-after pictures, there is probably more than one reason why. Maybe they don't have any happy patients who are willing to help them and allow their pictures to be shown. Maybe they don't have any good results to show you.

Those two reasons alone are enough to move on to the next candidate, because an experienced, talented surgeon has had plenty of patients with good outcomes. And when patients have good outcomes, they are almost always willing to let their picture be shown. I have hundreds of patients who have given their permission for me to show their pictures on the Internet, to my patients in the office, in my lectures to residents and medical students, and in the articles and publications I write. They are appreciative of a job well done. They are never paid or compensated in any way for letting me show their pictures. They do it out of the goodness of their hearts. **They** have done the hard work, not me. They have gone through the sacrifices and the recovery period, and they are proud of that. They're pleased with how they look and they want to help someone else achieve the same results.

If you were choosing a builder to construct your dream home, wouldn't you like to see a few of the other homes he has constructed? What would you think if he refused to show you any?

When requesting and viewing before-and-after pictures, keep these points in mind:

- Ask to see only un-retouched photos. Be on the lookout for any images that appear to be digitally enhanced.
- Compare the lighting and backgrounds of the two pictures. They should be the same in both.
- Compare makeup and hairstyles. Is the model wearing no makeup in the "before" shot, but wearing obvious makeup in the "after" photo? Is her hair a mess in the first one, but perfectly done in the second? Ideally, hair and makeup should be similar in both shots.
- If you are viewing photos of a neck lift or a facelift, is the model holding her head with her chin down in the

first one and her chin jutted out and lifted up in the second one? You can affect the anatomy and curvature of the neck or jawline (or even alter the appearance of the nose!) by angling the head in certain ways. If the model's head is not positioned the same way in both shots, something may be fishy.

In summary, if a surgeon is the least bit standoffish about showing pictures, or if the pictures you are shown are suspect in any way, that is grounds for serious suspicion. Thank them for their time and move on to the next.

Question 6: How do you choose which products (fillers, etc.) to carry?

The answer to this question *should* be, "I use only those products that bring about the best, longest-lasting, most natural-looking results for my patients." However, an unscrupulous doctor may be saying that, but secretly thinking, "I use only those products that earn me the highest profit margin when I use them." I always hope to goodness that's not the case, but unfortunately, sometimes it is.

When you ask this question, follow up by asking the doctor to point to some physiological reasons why they have chosen one product over another. Is this product better than another for fine lines on the surface of the skin? Is this one better for filling the deeper layers of the skin than the other product? Does this product provide longer lasting results than its competitor? Enquiring minds want to know.

And if you are being sold a product based solely upon its lower price point, beware. Usually the cost between competing products will vary by twenty to thirty percent at the most. Do not bargain shop when it comes to your face. Sure, you can go to a strip mall and visit a shop that just opened up last week, run by someone who went to a weekend course the month before, and she's offering two-syringes-for-the-price-of-one, or 75% off your first procedure. But if you come away from there looking deformed and you are forced to seek correction afterward with another surgeon, then that is the opposite of a bargain. That's what I call a rip off, and a dangerous one at that.

Also remember that these products (Botox or botulinum toxin injection, filler injection, cosmetic services, facials, peels and even surgery) are technique-dependent. You are not only paying for the product, but you are also paying for the expertise of the person who is administering it. When it comes to cosmetic procedures, you really do get what you pay for.

Question 7: Do you have a website? What is its purpose?

"Educating patients" should be the first answer. You should be able to gain some value from a surgeon's website. What can you learn here? Can you click a link and find specific information about the procedures offered through the clinic? Does the site show some legitimate before-and-after pictures? Are there phone numbers and email addresses to use if you have questions? Are you invited to ask questions even before you have scheduled a consultation? Is there a link to organizations in which that surgeon is a member or board certified?

All too often, company websites (no matter what type of business they're representing) are there for the ego of the person who put them there. *I am the greatest... Here are my awards... These are the hours we're open so you can come in and give me money... Here are the surgeries I do...* that type of thing. They'll list everything out in bullet points. That's a Me-Me-Me-type of website. That is not the way it ought to be.

For example, there should be bios of the surgeon and his or her teammates on the site so you can get to know more about them in advance of your visit. Remember, that surgeon will not be the one spending three, four, five hours with you in the weeks and days leading up to, and after, your surgery. It is just not possible. You will be relying on the other people in that practice. When you can learn more about them and even interact with them via the website (an eventually, over the phone and in person) that is a great thing.

Websites can serve to provide education for the patient, but of course the most important thing is the face-to-face meeting. Your surgery choices need to be based upon factual information coming in from unbiased sources. Remember that even the most professional-looking, informative surgeon's website is biased information to some extent. We don't spend $60,000 on those websites because they are fun to look at. Those sites are there to draw patients in. Never forget that this is a business and the website is a storefront. When you look at a website, you are looking at advertising. Judge everything you see with that in mind.

Question 8: Are you active in your community?

You will probably catch some surgeons off guard with this question. The first time a patient asked me this, I was caught way off guard. That's not necessarily a bad thing. This is an important question because if a physician really cares about you, then they probably care about other people, too. So when they say, "I really care about my patients," I think it is perfectly reasonable to reply by saying, "Great! So what kinds of caring things do you do in your community?" If he or

ws and doesn't have a quick, clear answer,
t that they don't care about people quite as
im to.

On the other hand, I would be reassured if that surgeon says, "I have a charitable organization of my own," or "I am active in my church," or "I love to spend time with my son's scout troop," or "I coach my daughter's soccer team on Saturdays," or "I serve on the board of our town's homeless shelter." Maybe they do mission trips, or offer their services at a free clinic. That is a physician who is a human being. That is a person who understands the human element; who understands that life sometimes deals folks a bad hand of cards. If you are frustrated after surgery, that doctor will be more likely to feel your pain. If you are very happy after surgery, that is a doctor who will celebrate with you.

Asking this question can teach you a lot about the surgeon as a person, and will help you learn more about their reputation within the community. That is excellent information to have.

Question 9: Have you ever been sued for malpractice?
You can either ask the surgeon directly, or go to www.mdnationwide.org to find out, or both. It is good for the patient to know if a surgeon they are considering has been

sued, but that information also has to be taken with a grain of salt. Every surgeon – even the best of the best – has had complications arise in their surgeries (more on this later) and since ours is a sue-happy nation, most surgeons have been named in a lawsuit at some point in their careers. Sometimes it is a legitimate case, other times, it is not.

Let me give you an example. A patient at a Veterans Hospital was planning to have eyelid surgery to correct obstruction of vision. He had a preoperative physical exam prior to surgery. Part of that exam was a screening chest x-ray, which showed an abnormality. The patient was notified and an appointment was made for him to see his primary care doctor for evaluation and a further work up. The patient chose not to keep that appointment with his primary care doctor. The eyelid surgery was done uneventfully and the patient was happy with the outcome.

Time marched on. The patient eventually was diagnosed with lung cancer after decades of smoking. He died. After his passing, his family sued Veterans Hospital for failing to adequately diagnose and treat his lung cancer earlier. Every doctor who cared for that patient was named in the suit. The Veterans Hospital settled the case, but each of those doctors is now listed in the National Practitioners Database as having settled a malpractice claim in the past.

Why am I giving you such a detailed example? Because the surgeon who did the eyelid surgery was me. Of course, I wish all that had not happened, but it did. So consider lawsuit information with a clear mind. Remember: having one traffic accident doesn't necessarily make someone a bad driver. A record with twenty car crashes on it may cause one to wonder, however.

BONUS QUESTION: You aren't going to make me look like (insert blatantly overdone celebrity name here), are you?

I put this question in here for entertainment purposes only. Please do not ask your surgeon this. People ask me this all the time. What answer are they expecting? Do they think any plastic surgeon with a brain cell would say yes? Of course not. We think those blatantly overdone celebrities look just as ridiculous as you think they do. Your surgeon has secondary gain in you looking great and natural when you're healed. If you are going to tell all your girlfriends about your surgery and who did it, rest assured your surgeon wants you to say positive things and refer your friends.

The celebrity train wrecks are products of unscrupulous check cashers who can't say no to a famous patient. We all know of the tragic loss of that talented recording artist known almost as much for his ever-shrinking nose as he was for his fantastic musical career. What he needed most was someone to care... to care more about him as a human being than they cared about money or for being part of the "entourage." He needed a doctor to say, "You need help! Let's cancel the concert and get you healthy again." He needed to be in a hospital and not on IV medication just to help him fall asleep in his own bedroom. The world lost a talented musical genius because doctors failed to make rational safe decisions.

The gossip magazines amaze me. Please do not use them as a reference for plastic surgery. They write cover stories on celebrity surgeries and make outlandish predictions of who has had what surgery. This is medical care we are talking about. The magazines hire doctors to claim they know what procedures these celebrities have had done. Imagine if Dr. Smarty McPompous was quoted in your weekly gossip magazine as saying, "I've personally never treated Ms. Glamour Girl, but I am sure she has had venereal disease and hemorrhoid surgery." You just cringed, didn't you? It's the same thing. That doctor is making assumptions about a patient's medical care. How they get away with that, I have no idea. But I see it all the time.

Some people just make bad decisions. Do your research and don't be one of them.

The Facility

I've had so much plastic surgery, when I die they will donate my body to Tupperware. Joan Rivers

Question 10: Is the facility where I would have my procedure accredited? If so, by which organization(s)?
Over the past decade, there have been a number of unfortunate incidents in which patients – including a couple of high profile people – died following surgeries conducted in settings unprepared for the complications that can and do occur with general anesthesia. Being prepared for those complications is what accreditation is all about.

Accreditation is a voluntary process in which health care facilities agree to adhere to a stringent set of patient care, safety, and quality standards. Independent accrediting agencies – most notably the Accreditation Association for Ambulatory Health Care (AAAHC) and The Joint Commission on Accreditation of Healthcare Organizations (JCAHO) – administer the accreditation process and conduct site visits to confirm that a health care facility has actually met and continues to meet those rigorous quality standards.

The vast majority of surgery centers that provide general anesthetic are accredited. Not all doctor's offices are, even when surgical procedures are performed there. If you are having a procedure with general anesthesia, *make certain that the facility where your procedure will be conducted has earned accreditation from a reputable agency, and that the accreditation is current.* I cannot stress this enough. Ask the surgeon or their support staff for the name of the facility's accrediting agency, and then follow up by calling the agency or checking its website to make sure the facility you are considering is in good standing. If it is, you can rest assured that the proper patient safety procedures and crisis plans are in place. If it is not in good standing for whatever reason, run to the nearest exit and don't look back. The life you save may be your own.

Question 11: At which hospital(s) do you have staff privileges for the procedure you will perform on me?
This question overlaps with a surgeon's board certification and education level. In order for a physician to have staff privileges at a hospital (in other words, to be able to bring in their patients and practice medicine there) they must apply in advance and prove that they meet the hospital's requirements. Generally speaking, they must be board certified (or board eligible) in the specialty for which they are providing services, demonstrate that they have completed a

Question 12: In the event of an emergency, what is the crisis plan?

If you have confirmed that the facility you are using is accredited for general anesthesia, then you can rest assured that there is a crisis plan already in place there, because facilities cannot achieve accreditation without one. Hopefully that crisis plan will never be used, but it sure is comforting to know it's there.

Ask the surgeon to describe the crisis plan to you. Ask if he/she has ever had to use it because of a complication. Every surgeon should be comfortable talking about complications. Why? Because every surgeon has had complications. Complications are learning experiences. There is not a doctor on earth who is completely immune from them. A surgeon who says he has never had a complication is either a liar, or in fact, not a surgeon at all.

You want to know that there is a recovery room – which is essentially a miniature intensive care unit – available in case of complications. Many surgery centers are attached to or are in close proximity to hospitals so if there is a problem, the patient can be quickly and efficiently transferred and cared for. Review the previous question about hospital privileges, and be sure your surgeon is affiliated with that nearby hospital.

Question 13: Do you have an in-office operating room? Why or why not?

There are pros and cons to both situations. On the plus side, in-office operating rooms are private. Your procedure will be done in a facility with which you're already familiar and comfortable. You are THE patient that day. You are not waiting in line behind a dozen others. You have the procedure done, you recover in the same place, and you go home. As long as it is a facility accredited for general anesthesia, staffed with experienced, board certified, nurturing health care providers and is near a hospital in case something goes wrong, an in-office operating room is a great environment in which to have a surgical procedure.

The downside to an in-office operating room is that it may not be accredited for general anesthesia. You may not have the high-powered equipment you'd find in a surgery center or hospital. There may be no a crisis plan in case of an emergency. This is best illustrated in real life terms by the unfortunate high profile cases in Florida and New York in which office procedures went horribly wrong, and patients lost their lives as a result.

Doctors who do not have in-office operating rooms see patients in their clinic and then do procedures at an outlying surgery center, or perhaps a hospital. The pros: the surgery center and hospital are larger. They are more accommodating to many different types of procedures.

There is greater flexibility with scheduling because of the large number of operating rooms they have. The disadvantages are that it may be less convenient than a one-stop shop, and also a bit more expensive. Surgery centers and hospitals have a motive for staying in business, and that is to make a profit. You will be charged accordingly.

The Support Team

Beauty is the illumination of your soul.
John O'Donohue

Question 14: Who is on your staff? What are their roles and qualifications? What can I expect from your support team?

The reality is that your surgeon will not be the one sitting with you for hours, holding your hand, calming your fears, and answering your routine phone calls. The surgeon's support team members – the receptionist, patient care coordinator, nurses, medical assistant, and other personnel – are the people you are actually going to spend the most time with before and after your procedure. These are the people you will rely upon the most for reassurance and answers to your questions and calls. They are the ones who will schedule your visits and procedures. They are the people who will help you with the nuts and bolts stuff; the dressings, drains, pains, and gains of surgery. In order to focus on what they do best – performing surgery – surgeons who are busy and in demand have no choice but to delegate these sorts of less specialized tasks to their teammates.

That is not a bad thing. The more qualified people you have supporting you as a patient, the better.

For example, I have a nurse, medical assistant, patient care coordinator, and other people in the office to assist my patients and me. From your perspective, meeting those people beforehand is critical. Finding out what they are like in advance and knowing that you can call on them if you have a question is very reassuring. You don't have to wait for the surgeon to call you back at the end of the day to ask simple questions when the support team is ready, willing and able to assist you.

So the bottom line is that the support team is the engine that makes the office run. The people working alongside the surgeon help her be more efficient at what she does. Surgery is a team effort. Meeting each member of the team beforehand and knowing who they are and what they do is important to your health and your peace of mind.

Question 15: Can I call or email questions to someone in your office? If so, whom?

Who is going to be your main point of contact among the team members? Maybe it is the surgeon. Perhaps it is a head nurse or medical assistant. Identify the person in charge of answering your questions so you will know exactly whom to call if the need arises.

One caveat, though: too many calls will get you in trouble, no matter which person you are calling. There is a fine line between (1) having a legitimate concern, and (2) calling every three hours for reassurance. Those are two different things, having a question and simply seeking a hand to hold. Your surgeon and support team should be willing to offer that hand to some extent, but you have to take ultimate responsibility for your own care.

Please allow me to offer you a pearl of wisdom at this point that will make your experience at the surgeon's office much more pleasant: BE NICE! If you are abrasive, pompous and rude to the support staff, you are just making it more difficult for them to help you. Sorry to break it to you, but it's true: kind, grateful patients get more attentive care. That's just the way it is. If you are mean to the people who check you in and take your history, believe me, your surgeon will know about it before she even sees you. If you walk into the clinic with a green face and a pointy hat and you are angry about a house recently falling on your sister, don't expect us munchkins to line up to help you. We will be hiding behind the flowers!

During my residency (almost two decades ago at the time of writing this book) I had the opportunity to spend a day with a well-known facial plastic surgeon in Beverly Hills. Through the course of the morning we were in and out of surgical cases and met with a few follow-up patients in clinic.

Within a total of four hours, the surgeon's personal assistant brought him five different phone messages, all from the same patient. He answered each with a call back and there was no problem or reason for concern in any of them. On the fifth message delivery, he turned to me and held the message to reveal the name of a famous movie actress. He looked at me forlornly and said, "It doesn't matter who they are. Anyone can be a pain-in-the-ass if they want to."

Remember: everything in moderation.

I recall one patient who called my office 21 times in a 72-hour post-operative period. How do I know that? Because every time you call a medical office and speak with a health care provider, that communication is documented. Your question, and the answer you were given, is documented. So if you want to play games and ask three different people in the office the same question in hopes of finding a different answer, they very likely already know you've called before. Believe me, a doctor's office has no secondary gain in giving you an unsafe answer. They want you to have a great outcome, too. They do have secondary gain in happy, healthy patients.

You have to take ultimate responsibility for your own recovery. You are the patient. You chose to have this surgery. Participate in your recovery. Participate in the wound care. Read the instructions before surgery and read them again afterward, and then follow them. If the directions provided are good and you follow them, it is unlikely that you will need to call in at all.

The Cost

Beauty is a sign of intelligence.

Andy Warhol

Question 16: Will insurance cover any of the costs associated with my plastic surgery?

First of all, allow me to reiterate that bargain shopping for your face and body is not something I ever recommend. Sometimes you do get what you pay for. Sometimes quality does correspond with price, but not always. I'm not going to say that all of the most expensive surgeons in the world are the best. Just because one has a plastic surgery practice in Beverly Hills doesn't mean one is any good. Just look at the mangled faces of several Hollywood stars for the unfortunate proof of that.

Now, about insurance. The basis for whether or not insurance covers a plastic surgery procedure has to do with function and dysfunction. It has to do with whether or not some bodily feature is causing an actual physical problem. For example, if the upper eyelids are blocking someone's vision and making it unsafe for them to drive, or causing headaches from them having to hold their brows up all day, then in many cases, upper eyelid blepharoplasty can be covered by insurance. If a person's nose is crooked from a car accident or a previous injury and they simply can't breathe through it very well, then reconstruction and straightening of that nose would likely be covered by insurance. But if the person is seeking to have that nose look different than it did before the injury, then that would be *cosmetic* surgery. If a woman's breasts are so big that they are causing her to experience back, shoulder or neck pain; or if her bra straps are digging into her skin, then breast reduction may be covered by insurance because it is correcting a functional problem in order to improve her health. But if it's just because she wants her breasts to be smaller so she can fit into a different size dress, then that is *cosmetic* surgery. Cosmetic surgery done on insurance time and with insurance payment has a name, and it is **fraud**. No ethical doctor will be willing to do that.

To bend the rules just to get insurance to pay for something is to walk a very treacherous line. Stay away from that line. Patients can be just as guilty of insurance fraud as doctors, so if you are trying to have insurance pay for your purely cosmetic surgery, you are committing fraud. You are breaking the law. Don't put yourself and your family in that kind of jeopardy.

Question 17: What about the costs not covered by insurance? How does that work? What are my payment options?

First of all, you can expect to hand over a deposit of anywhere from ten to fifty percent of the cost of the surgery in order to schedule your procedure. This is because it costs the surgeon money to reserve time for you. When a surgeon blocks surgery time, it means that not only is he reserving that operating room, but he also is reserving specialized equipment that will be sterilized and ready upon his arrival. He is reserving an entire team, including an anesthesia doctor, to be there on that day, mobilized specifically to care for you. If you don't pay anything in advance and then decide to cancel the day before the surgery, you have just cost that surgeon a lot of money. As much as we don't like to talk about it, we surgeons are in business, too. We have mortgages and expenses to pay, just like you. So expect to shell out a deposit to schedule your procedure, and then count on paying the remainder prior to the day of surgery.

Some patients balk at having to pay in advance. If you are one of them, think of it this way: even though you get to make installment payments for years after buying a car from your local dealership, that dealer was actually paid in full before you drove the car off the lot. A financing company paid off your car on day one, and your after-the-fact payments go to them. It's the same thing at the grocery store. You don't walk out of the market with a cart full of groceries saying, "I'll pay for these later!" No, you pay in advance, before using any of the products in that cart.

Cosmetic surgery is exactly the same. You pay before you have that procedure done. The payment covers the expertise of the surgeon and the team. It covers the surgery itself. It covers the sutures, the dressings and the drains that are in place afterward. It covers the follow up visits, and the questions over the phone.

Just like when you purchase a car from a dealer, financing is available to help you if you don't have enough money saved up for the whole thing. Some physicians offer their own in-house financing, but most don't. If yours doesn't, you can use a regular credit card to pay for the procedure, or you can get help from a special health care financing program. Three of the better known programs are:

Care Credit (www.CareCredit.com)
My Medical Loan (www.MyMedicalLoan.com)
My Medical Financing (www.MyMedicalFinancing.com)

Applying for this type of financing is like applying for a credit card. Remember, these financing programs are separate from your surgery provider. They pay the surgeon in advance, and you make monthly payments to them afterward – with interest, of course. If you fail to make payments to the financing company, it will take action to collect them, and it will do so aggressively. Don't get mad at your surgeon if you have failed to make payments to a financing company and they are seeking payment. That arrangement is between you and your financing company, and it is a decision you made. Do the right thing.

Other financing options include bank loans, home equity loans or lines of credit, or loans from your 401(k). Think about it – most folks don't even blink when it comes to using loans to refurbish their kitchen, purchase a new car, or help pay for their or their child's education. There is nothing inherently wrong with using a loan to improve the way you look and feel for the rest of your life. It can be a very good thing – but only as long as you are not living beyond your means or otherwise overextending yourself. Just as you should not buy a car that you can't afford, you should not have cosmetic surgery if you can't afford it.

Instead of borrowing, save up the money yourself, or ask your family and friends for donations to your Tummy Tuck Fund in lieu of holiday or birthday gifts this year. Why not? It sure beats another ugly sweater under the tree on Christmas morning!

Question 18: Is there a charge for consultations?

I estimate that roughly half of surgeons offer complimentary consultations. They do that for one reason: to entice more people to come in and talk to them. The downside of this approach is that surgeons who schedule complimentary consultations have twice as many no-shows as those who charge fees.

Generally speaking, a surgeon who charges a fee for consultation is in higher demand. That's just Keynesian economics in action; it's a matter of supply and demand. If they have the ability to charge for a consultation, then there is probably a healthy demand for those consultations. As a patient, I wouldn't balk at all if there were a consultation fee. In fact, I would expect it. You are not paying only for the doctor's time; you are also paying for their expert opinion, and for the learning that results from spending time discussing your unique situation with them. Paying a $150 consultation fee and sitting down with the doctor who's willing to answer all your questions, make recommendations for what type of surgery they think is best for you, show you before and after pictures, give a quote for that surgery, provide written and visual information on what to expect before, during and after the procedure and then give you the opportunity to meet with a patient care coordinator who will discuss payment and scheduling options – well, that is money well-spent, wouldn't you agree?

However, if you paid a $150 consultation fee and only got to talk to the doctor for thirty seconds, then that is not a good deal. So when you call to set up a paid consultation, ask for an explanation of what you can expect during your visit. Find out how much time you'll be able to spend with the surgeon and other support team members. If you don't like what you hear, move on to the next doctor on your list.

Question 19: If I need a touch-up procedure or revision, who pays for it?

Unfortunately, touchups and revisions are quite common in the cosmetic surgery business. Cosmetic surgery is an art, not an exact science. The human body doesn't always heal exactly as one would expect every single time. If something is a bit disappointing in your outcome – perhaps a visual defect like one side being considerably different than the other – the surgeon might suggest a touchup or a revision procedure. The payment for these differs from practice to practice. In my practice, the payment is for the procedure **and** the outcome, so whatever it takes to make my patient happy (within reason) is included in the original price.

That may not always be the case with other surgeons. You may be expected to pay for follow up procedures and revisions. If you have a breast augmentation and one breast forms capsular contracture afterwards and it becomes necessary to go back in and revise that, you may have to pay for the surgeon, the anesthesiologist and the facility all over again, and that may be a significant expense that you didn't anticipate. This is why it is important to ask about the doctor's revision and touchup policy in advance. If they say they don't cover any revisions or complications afterwards, then at least you will be somewhat prepared when you get hit with a bill for further work.

And here's another news flash: in most cases, complications from cosmetic surgery are not covered by insurance. That means that if you have a heart attack during cosmetic surgery and you are admitted to the intensive care unit, your insurance probably is not going to pay for that. The insurance company's position is that, since you chose to take the risk of undergoing surgery, they should not have to cover any of the resulting fallout. In my opinion, that is unfortunate and downright wrong. A guy can get drunk and drive off the bridge, and insurance will pay for him to be in the intensive care unit on a ventilator for the rest of his life. But if I choose to improve my eyelids and there is a complication that requires a procedure afterward, insurance won't cover it? There is no logic in that. There is a bias against cosmetic surgery. Therefore, you can expect zero insurance coverage for any complications arising from it. Just one more reason to proceed with caution, and choose the best surgeon you can find.

The Consultation

You can be gorgeous at thirty, charming at forty, and irresistible for the rest of your life. Coco Chanel

Question 20: What happens in a consultation?

A consultation is essentially an opportunity for the physician and the patient to meet and communicate. When you meet someone for the first time – say, in a grocery store or at your child's school – your initial impression is formed within the first ten seconds. The same thing occurs for the patient and the surgeon in the early moments of a consultation. If the surgeon is positive, outgoing, smiling and making eye contact, then that is a good sign. If the patient is positive, outgoing, smiling and making eye contact, then you've got a great start to a relationship, no matter what the context.

But remember: this is a medical appointment. As much as you would like to talk exclusively about the actual procedure and how it's going to make you look and feel better, that person in front of you is still a doctor who is required to provide medical care. Therefore, you can expect to be weighed and have your temperature, blood pressure and pulse checked – all the things you would expect at a normal doctor's office. A nurse or medical assistant is going to ask you about medications, allergies and adverse reactions to anesthesia in the past. They're going to ask about your past medical history, especially previous surgeries. It is absolutely vital to be completely open and honest about that. I have had many patients who were too embarrassed to divulge that they'd had a previous operation performed on them. Only at the time of surgery did I find out that they'd had a rhinoplasty before but had neglected to tell me about it. That not only affects the surgical plan and the safety of the current procedure; it can also change the surgical outcome. So be completely honest about any work you have had done in the past.

Also, be honest about your social habits – especially about smoking, alcohol consumption and other drug use. I am not going to get up on a soapbox about vices. We all have them. I have them, too. But when it comes to something as serious as surgery, you have to be open and honest about your habits because they can make the procedure unsafe and affect the outcome. Don't be bashful about it. Believe me, we've heard it all before and we will not judge you. Anything you say is confidential; that's the law.

Expect to see some of the before-and-after photos we covered earlier. Expect to spend time with the surgeon (and perhaps also a physician's assistant, nurse or medical assistant) asking any questions you want to ask. I think the best medical professionals are the ones who want to educate their patients about **why** they are making a particular recommendation. Expect to receive solid, instructive answers. If you don't understand, ask. If you can't see, stop. Those are just basic tenets in life. If you are in a consultation and you don't understand something, don't just smile and nod. There are no extra credit points for being cool. Just ask if you don't understand.

Expect to have several photos taken. These are not glamour shots. These are not for publication. They are medical documentation of what you looked like before surgery; they establish a baseline, so to speak. Later on, you and your surgeon will be able to look back at those pictures and track your progress. These pictures are held in the strictest confidentiality. That's the law, too. They are only shown to others if you sign a permission form.

Finally, at the time of consultation you will likely receive a quote for the cost of your procedure. Usually, you will get this from a patient care coordinator or another person in a similar role who will write out all the projected expenses involved in your case and sit down to discuss it with you. Not only will that include the surgeon's fee, but it may also include the facility, the equipment, medications, anesthesiologist, etc.

In summary, the consultation with the surgeon and staff is critical to a procedure's success, yet many patients and surgeons are woefully unprepared for it. When you have a surgeon who spends a grand total of ninety seconds in the room – with his hand on the doorknob the whole time – and who then says, "So that's what I suggest we do. See you on the big day. Thanks..." and walks out before you have a chance to ask any questions, there is a huge gap between what you know and what you need to know. If you ever feel as if you're being put off as a patient, my suggestion is get up and walk toward the door, because you are the buyer in this transaction. The ball is in your court.

Question 21: How do you know that I am candidate for the procedure I am requesting (or that you are recommending)? What are my alternatives?

First, let me say that we plastic surgeons are not in the surgery business. We are in the "make people feel better about themselves" business. If that means clarifying for a patient that I would not suggest doing anything – that they look great and that their contours are beautiful – and they leave my office feeling better about themselves, confident that they have made a sound decision to not have an unnecessary surgery, then I have done my job well.

That said, your possible treatments range from doing nothing to undergoing the most aggressive, game changing surgery we have to offer, and everything in between. So while you may come into a consultation convinced that you need a particular surgery, you may learn that you can achieve a happy result with a more conservative approach like injectable filler, botulinum toxin, or better skincare. A surgeon does not necessarily have to do surgery. The best surgeons know when **not** to operate. I talk people out of surgery all the time, because sometimes surgery is not the best option for them.

My advice is to ask the above question and *really listen with an open mind* to the surgeon's response. You may learn about a terrific option you never even considered before. Always get a second or third opinion if you have any doubts whatsoever about the surgeon's recommendation.

Question 22: Can I show you pictures of what I want?
Pictures are a double-edged sword. On the one hand, I've had women walk in with photos of Ashlee Simpson and request that I give them her chin. I had one gentlemen hand me a picture of Ricky Martin and declare, "I want this nose."

Whenever that happens, my response goes something like this: "You are a fine looking person, but you are not Ashlee Simpson. You are not Ricky Martin. You don't have their parents. Your DNA is different than theirs. Your collagen is different than theirs, and so are your bones. I'm sorry to break it to you, but you probably cannot have Brad

Pitt's nose or Cate Blanchett's cheekbones either. It doesn't work that way."

That said, as long as you are showing reasonable pictures and your expectations are realistic, seeing pictures can help the surgeon gain some insight into what you're seeking. Before handing over any pictures, try putting it this way to your surgeon: "Could I show you some examples of what I'm thinking? I realize I'm not this person, but I am hoping to move in this general direction." Be as specific as you can. If you say to your hairstylist, "I want my hair shorter..." do you mean you want a half inch taken off or do you want your head shaved? I know, I know. That is an extreme example, but you get the idea. Showing her photos of the hairstyle you are seeking is often very helpful. The same applies to cosmetic plastic surgery.

Your surgeon should have no problem with that approach – in fact, she should welcome it.

Question 23: Who will my consultation be with – a physician's assistant (PA) or the actual surgeon?
Do not wait until you arrive at the surgeon's office before asking this question. Inquire about this when you call to schedule your consultation, because the answer may compel you to skip that particular doctor altogether.

I've heard of practices in which the patient doesn't meet their surgeon until the day of their procedure. In some instances, patients do not see the surgeon at all. I am not a fan of that. As healthcare providers, we need to provide care. That means meeting our patients beforehand, listening to them and working with them to create a customized plan for their care and treatment. If a surgeon doesn't work that way, you can choose to seek care elsewhere, or at least know what to expect in advance.

But in most consultations, you can expect to meet a medical assistant, nurse or physician's assistant first for a review of your medical history and a physical exam prior to meeting the surgeon. Or you may come in for a free or lower priced consultation with the physician's assistant or nurse, and then move on to another consultation with the surgeon at a later date.

Sometimes that's a helpful approach because it allows the surgeon's office to weed out people who may not be surgical candidates, or who may not want surgery once they learn more about it. It can also be good for you as a patient because you can learn about other options without paying an expensive fee to see the surgeon. Still, I recommend that you definitely talk with your surgeon before scheduling your procedure and paying any money, just in case the two of you are not a good match.

Question 24: I am a smoker. Will you perform surgery on me?

The answer is yes and no. If you are a person who smokes two packs a day and you are not going to quit, expect to hear a no. As stated earlier, first and foremost, your surgeon is a doctor. She is there to care for you and to make sure that you are safe. If you smoke like a chimney, it can greatly affect the outcome of the surgery and it can greatly affect your safety. If a surgeon is willing to take those kinds of risks and cut those kinds of corners just because a patient is willing to write a check, then that is probably a surgeon you ought to reject. Move on and seek another opinion.

Now, if someone smokes an occasional cigarette but they are truly committed to having the surgery, in many cases they will be able to commit to quitting smoking. I see it happen all the time. If you are truly dedicated to getting your very best outcome, you should be willing to do that. You should be willing to make sacrifices like changing your diet, using some supplements that will help you heal, backing off on smoking, and slowing down on drinking.

You may say that you are truly committed to your best outcome, yet you don't want to quit smoking. OK, that's fine. That just means that you are *not* truly committed to your best outcome. You are addicted.

I have many patients who will back off smoking two weeks before surgery. A week or two afterward, we tell them that if they choose to return to smoking, they can do so. In many cases, we find that these people will have lost their desire to smoke. They have come to realize how much better things can be without it, and how much money they can save. That's not to say they never have that jones; that urge to light up again. But more often than not, they come to appreciate all the positive benefits they have received from quitting, and they discover that smoking cessation was easier and more rewarding than they ever imagined.

Now I will tell you a little secret that all of us doctors want you to know. **Smoking is bad for you; don't do it.** If you don't believe that, send your book back to me. I'll refund your money and you can put it toward your future medical expenses.

Question 25: What is digital imaging? How realistic is it?
Digital imaging is taking a patient's photograph and using computer software to alter the image so it shows a reasonable expectation of the surgical outcome. We can change the shape, contours, coloration, or other elements in the picture of the person's face or body to represent what we believe we can achieve with surgery or some other procedure. For example, it works great to show a rhinoplasty patient what they might look like with the nasal hump reduced. In many cases, we take those digitally altered

images into the operating room and refer to them during surgery as reminders of the goal we are seeking for that patient.

While digital imaging has been a wonderful aid in cosmetic surgery, it can also be used misleadingly to promote certain procedures or products. I see it sometimes in advertising photos. In my opinion, it should never be utilized as a selling tool. It is an educational tool to show someone what a reasonable, approximated result could be.

Digital imaging is becoming more popular with each passing day, but there remain many offices that do not use it at all. That is perfectly fine. Some surgeons don't want to risk giving a false impression or doing anything that could mislead anyone in any way. That is understandable, but I think it is a terrific tool as long as it is used responsibly. Always, always, always remember that a digital image is nothing more than an estimate. It is a hopeful prediction of an outcome. It is not a guarantee.

And, by the way, all those models you see in fashion magazines? Lots of digital imaging happening there. You are beautiful just the way you are. Strive to be the best YOU can be, not to be someone else.

Question 26: Can I talk to any of your previous patients?
Although cosmetic surgery is a private matter, surgeons who are excellent at their craft tend to have lots of happy patients, and some of those patients will always be willing to share their experience with others for the purpose of helping them make informed decisions.

For instance, I have a number of patients who have volunteered to talk to other folks who are considering the same kind of procedure they had. I did not even have to ask. These are men and women who are delighted with their outcomes and have offered to help others by answering their questions from a patient's perspective. We take them up on that offer all the time. These generous individuals make it possible for a prospective patient to call them from the comfort and security of their home and ask questions of someone who has actually been down this road before. It is a wonderful thing. It's so wonderful that you might want to consider sending a thank you note. Who knows? You may gain a new friend.

Most surgeons who are skilled at what they do have a list of people who will share their stories with others. So if you ask this question and you get a refusal from your surgeon, take that under advisement, so to speak.

Question 27: There are so many marketing gimmicks for various procedures. How can I cut through all the clutter to find what really works?

You are correct: the cosmetic surgery business is becoming more and more commoditized every day. In some cases, truth in advertising has been sacrificed completely in favor of the almighty dollar. This is terribly unfortunate. It should not come down to the best *marketed* surgery. It should come down to the best surgery, period.

The same is true with skincare products. Just because something has a glossy container, costs a lot of money and is promoted by a celebrity does not mean it works. Trust me when I tell you that many of those products are nothing more than the equivalent of what you can buy at the corner drugstore for a few bucks. The only differences are the glossy container, the astronomical price point and the high-powered person's endorsement.

Do not be fooled by gimmicks. Do not be dazzled by slick sales pitches. To find the product or procedure that will work best for you, clear your head and do a deep dive to get past the hype. Products that are effective are backed by clinical research that proves it. Products that work are usually warranted to work. Ask the skin care expert or dermatologist helping you what she uses. That's usually the strongest endorsement. Find respected experts you can trust, and ask a lot of questions. Find real people who have had that same procedure or used that same product, and inquire about their experience. Ask about what to expect; what the possible outcomes can be. Investigate the indications, risks, complications and alternatives for any procedure or product you are thinking about using. Apply the same good judgment and practice the same due diligence you would employ if you were thinking about ordering that procedure or product for the person you love the most in your life.

Take your time, use common sense, and always remember: **if it seems too good to be true, it probably is.**

Question 28: What current habits do I need to change to ensure that I am in the best health and cleared to undergo surgery?

Smoking, high doses of caffeine, drug and alcohol abuse, poor nutrition, stress, a sedentary lifestyle and a lack of sleep can all affect a patient's surgical outcomes in an adverse fashion. For example, heavy alcohol use can affect your liver and therefore the clotting of your blood, making you bruise and bleed more easily. High caffeine intake can raise blood pressure and cause withdrawal symptoms, such as headaches and agitation, when you can't have caffeine early after surgery. A slow metabolism stemming from poor nutrition and a lack of sleep or exercise negatively affects post-op healing. An unhealthy response to stress plays a huge role in inhibiting your immune system.

On the other hand, a patient with an active metabolism who exercises and deals effectively with stress, has a healthy diet, takes appropriate supplements and decreases toxins is a patient who heals more quickly and efficiently. That's just a fact.

So expect to receive a lengthy list of things to do and things to avoid leading up to your surgery date. Prepare yourself to follow the doctor's orders to the letter, or you may find yourself disappointed when your surgeon refuses to operate on you. Those orders are there for your own health and safety.

Question 29: I've just had a bad breakup (or other major life disappointment), and I think having plastic surgery will help get me over it. Do you think cosmetic interventions can have an impact on the quality of life?
Plastic surgery changes physical attributes like skin, muscle, cartilage and bone – but it does not change emotions. So the short answer is no; cosmetic surgery will not get you over your breakup.

Now, I say that tempered with the fact that when you change the way you look for the better, you feel better about yourself. That's why people have cosmetic surgery in the first place. I will say it again: I am not in the surgery business. I am in the "make people feel better about themselves" business. If feeling better about yourself helps you to be more confident in a job interview, in interactions with a person to whom you are attracted, in just living your daily life, then yes, absolutely it helps. But to use cosmetic surgery as a panacea for freeing yourself of the pain of a broken relationship, or thinking of it as a guarantee that you will meet the mate of your dreams? That's just wishful thinking. Happiness in life is all about the whole. It is not about any one aspect of yourself. You must strive to do what is best for each aspect to benefit the whole.

For example, you may ask yourself: *Is it really the awkward shape of my nose that is bothering me, or is it the domestic abuse that caused it?* I can change your broken nose, but I cannot change the fact that it was your ex-husband who caused it. That truth can be frustrating for a surgeon and it can be frustrating for a patient. In cases like that, sometimes the right choice is not having surgery at all – or at least putting it off until you can make your decision based on a more constructive criteria. A responsible surgeon who has your best interests at heart will recommend that type of conservative approach every time.

As for cosmetic surgery's impact on your quality of life in general: in our society, people who are more attractive get more opportunities. It's true. Research backs it up – that's just the way it is. Occupations, advancements, relationships with others – all are impacted by one's appearance and self-esteem. Cosmetic surgery can and does make life better. That is why you are choosing to do it. And by the way, this must be your decision and no one else's. If you are doing it for a husband who thinks you need a breast augmentation, or for an agent who thinks you need a smaller nose in order to be successful, then those are not the right reasons. **You** are the person who has to put on a bra over those augmented breasts, not your husband. **You** are the person who has to look at that nose in the mirror every morning, not your agent. Deciding to have cosmetic surgery can absolutely have benefits, but that decision must be made for the right reason.

Doing it for yourself is the ONLY right reason.

Pre-Op

I don't plan to grow old gracefully. I plan to have face-lifts until my ears meet.
Rita Rudner

Question 30: What medications and herbal or holistic supplements should I stop/start prior to surgery?

It is absolutely necessary that your doctor and the nursing staff prior to surgery specifically clear all of your current medications. The use of some medications must be discontinued as much as two weeks before your surgery date. Your surgeon should be able to provide you with a list of medications and supplements that you should and should not take leading up to your procedure. Remember: the list is only a guideline. It is not all-inclusive. If you have questions about your medications, ask!

MEDICATIONS TO AVOID BEFORE AND AFTER SURGERY

If you are taking any medications on this list, they should be discontinued two weeks prior to surgery and only acetaminophen should be taken for pain. All other medications that you are currently taking must be specifically cleared by your doctor prior to surgery. These lists are recommendations only and may be used as a guideline. They are not all inclusive lists. It is absolutely necessary that all of your current medications be specifically cleared by your doctor and the nursing staff prior to surgery. These medications may be resumed two weeks following surgery. If you have questions about your medications, ask!

ASPIRIN MEDICATIONS TO AVOID

4-Way Cold Tabs
5-Aminosalicyclic Acid
Acetylsalicylic Acid
Adprin-B products
Alka-Seltzer products
Amigesic
Anacin products
Anexsia w/Codeine
Argesic-SA
Arthra-G
Arthriten products
Arthritis Foundation products
Arthritis Pain formula
Arthritis Strength BC Powder
Arthropan
ASA
Asacol
Ascriptin products
Aspergum
Asprimox products
Axotal
Azdone
Azulfidine products
B-A-C
Backache Maximum Strength Relief

Bayer Products
BC Powder
Bismatrol products
Buffered Aspirin
Bufferin products
Carisoprodol Compound
Cheracol
Choline Magnesium Trisalicylate
Choline Salicylate
Cope
Coricidin
Cortisone Medications
Damason-P
Darvon Compound – 65
Darvon/ASA
Dipentum
Disalcid
Doan's products
Dolobid
Dristan
Duragesic
Easprin
Ecotrin products
Empirin products
Equagesic
Excedrin products
Fiorgen PF
Fiorinal products
Gelpirin

Genprin
Gensan
Goody's Extra Strength Headache Powders
Halfprin products
Magnaprin products
Norgesic products
Norwich products
Olsalazine
Orphengesic products
Percodan products
Robaxisal
Rowasa
Roxiprin
Saleto products
Salflex
Salicylate products
Salsalate Salsitab
Scot-Tussin Original 5-Action
Sine-off Sinutab Sodium
Salicylate Sodol Compound
Soma Compound
St. Joseph Aspirin
Vanquish
Wesprin
Willow Bark products
Zorprin

IBUPROFEN MEDICATIONS TO AVOID

Actron Acular (ophthalmic)
Advil products
Aleve
Anaprox products
Ansaid
Cataflam
Clinoril
Daypro
Diclofenac
Dimetapp Sinus
Dristan Sinus
Etodolac
Feldene
Fenoprofen
Flurbiprofen
Genpril
Indocin products
Indomethacin products
Ketoprofen
Ketorolac
Lodine
Meclofenamate
Meclomen
Mefenamic Acid
Menadol
Midol products
Motrin products
Nabumetone
Nalfon products
Naprelan
Naprosyn products
Naprox X
Naproxen
Nuprin
Ocufen (ophthalmic)
Orudis products
Oruvail
Oxaprozin
Piroxicam
Ponstel
Profenal
Relafen
Rhinocaps
Sine-Aid products
Sulindac
Suprofen
Tolectin products
Tolmetin
Toradol
Voltaren

OTHER MEDICATIONS TO AVOID

Acutrim
Actifed
Anexsia
Anisindione
Anturane Arthritis
Bufferin BC Tablets
Children's Advil
Clinoril C
Contac
Coumadin
Dalteparin injection
Dicumarol
Dipyridamole
Doxycycline
Emagrin
Enoxaparin injection
Fish Oil Capsules
Flagyl
Fragmin injection
Furadantin
Garlic
Heparin
Hydrocortisone
Isollyl
Lovenox injection
Macrodantin
Mellaril
Miradon
Opasal Pan-PAC
Pentoxifylline
Persantine
Phenylpropanolamine
Prednisone (unless ok'd by your surgeon)
Stelazine
Sulfinpyrazone
Tenuate
Tenuate Dospan
Thorazine
Ticlid
Ticlopidine
Trental
Ursinus
Vibramycin
Vitamin E
Warfarin
Tricyclic

ANTIDEPRESSANT MEDICATIONS TO AVOID

Adapin
Amitriptyline
Amoxapine
Anafranil
Asendin
Aventyl
Clomipramine
Desipramine
Doxepin
Elavil
Endep
Etrafon products
Imipramine
Janimine
Limbitrol products
Ludiomil
Maprotiline
Norpramin
Nortriptyline
Pamelor
Pertofrane
Protriptyline
Sinequan
Surmontil
Tofranil
Triavil
Vivactil

HERBAL MEDICATIONS TO AVOID

Ginkgo Biloba
Ginseng
St. John's Wort

Question 31: On the day of my surgery, who will evaluate me?

You will likely have contact with a number of people who are each charged with checking and confirming specific things to ensure that all the medical and legal ducks are in a row.

First, you can expect to undergo an intake process. The legal ramifications of having surgery are overwhelming, and so is the paperwork required to document it. The person doing your intake is not handing you all of those papers and telling you all of those things because it is fun for them to sit there explaining the same piece of paper over and over again every day. It's just that the regulations and requirements for surgery centers are extensive, and they all have to be addressed. Expect to sign a lot of forms. Also be prepared to make any final payments before passing GO.

Next, you will move on to a nurse or a medical assistant who is going to ask you a series of questions they already really know the answers to. They are going to ask, "What procedure are you having done today?" "What meds do you take?" "What are you allergic to?" They are only confirming and checking boxes to make sure that every single base has been covered. If you are there to have your nose fixed and you end up with larger breasts when you wake up from anesthesia, that may fall into the "less than ideal" category, if you know what I mean.

After that's done, you will probably meet with the anesthesia provider, be it an anesthesiologist or a nurse anesthetist. They will ask you more medical history questions, and discuss your previous reactions to anesthesia. They will also explain the process of anesthesia and tell you about some of the medications that will be used.

You should then expect to meet with your surgeon prior to anesthesia. She may draw lines on your face or body, which will serve as references during your procedure. While you may feel like a whiteboard or an *Etch A Sketch* screen, remember that these drawings are there for your safety and to help the surgeon provide the very best results.

Let me reassure you about the moments before your surgery. If you are nervous and anxious, you are perfectly normal. Every patient is to some extent before surgery. Everyone you meet is specifically there to care for you. They are on your side. Know that your anxiety is a normal emotional defense mechanism. Just knowing that in advance will help you feel more at ease.

Intake can be a long, exhaustive process, but that attention to detail can make the difference between a bad outcome and a good outcome. Be patient. (No pun intended.)

The Procedure

Beauty lasts five minutes. Maybe longer if you have a good plastic surgeon.

Tia Carrere

Question 32: Who will administer my anesthesia?
That can vary. If it is a limited procedure using a very low level of sedation in the office, the nurse may administer your anesthesia. Anesthesia may be administered orally or through an intravenous line. General anesthesia is provided either by a nurse anesthetist or an anesthesiologist. The law requires that an anesthesia provider is with you and monitoring you constantly from the moment you go to sleep until the time you wake up.

Find out if your surgeon has an anesthesia provider on his team, or if he uses the services of an anesthesia group – a private practice that provides nurse anesthetists and anesthesiologists for doctors performing surgery at a local surgery center or hospital. If you are familiar with the

anesthesia group and already have a specific prov
mind that you know and trust, in most cases you are allowed
to request that person for your procedure. It is up to your
anesthesia provider whether or not he or she will honor that
request, however. Inquire well in advance so there will be no
surprises on game day.

Question 33: What are my options for anesthesia, and what are the associated risks?

The first option for anesthesia is to not have any at all. Some minor procedures in the office are done without it, or with local anesthesia like you would get at a dentist's office. The removal of moles, small cysts or skin tags, as well as most injectable fillers, can be carried out with minimal or no anesthesia. Other procedures can be done with a more powerful local anesthesia while the patient is completely awake. We often combine local anesthesia with a varying level of sedation – perhaps a little Valium to take the edge off – all the way up to an IV sedative that makes you go to sleep and wake up later having little or no memory of the procedure. Most chest and body procedures and some facial procedures are done with complete general anesthesia. Your airway and breathing are safely controlled by your anesthesiologist and you are heavily monitored throughout the procedure. It really depends on the case and how invasive the surgery is going to be.

Anesthesia impacts the systems of your body and your organs, such as your heart, lungs, liver and kidney function. Adverse reactions to the anesthetic agents are exceedingly rare, but they can be fatal if not addressed and managed properly. Risks, while rare and drastic, include stroke, heart attack and death. You can expect to see those three things on every consent form, because even though they are atypical, they can and do occur. People often refer to these kinds of bad outcomes as a one-in-a-million kind of risk. That's fine. Just remember that every week, somebody wins the lottery somewhere… and that's a one-in-a-million chance, too. You have to understand exactly what you're getting into.

Question 34: Will someone monitor me throughout my procedure? If so, who?

Over the past few decades, the surgical monitoring process has improved dramatically. These days we can keep tabs on practically every physiological function a patient has during surgery, no matter how minor or major the procedure may be.

If you are having only a mild sedative as described at the beginning of the previous question, it may be the nurse who monitors you and keeps a close eye on your vital signs. But if you are having general anesthetic or an anesthesia procedure at an accredited surgery center, an anesthesia provider is required to be with you every moment of your case. Again, there are strict monitoring regulations regarding that, and that's a good thing.

You want to make certain that some sort of medical professional will be there to keep an eye on you the whole time, no matter what the procedure. So do not hesitate to ask your surgeon for details about that. Her answer should ease your mind. If it doesn't, mark that one in the "con" column of your T-Chart of pros and cons.

Question 35: What will be my experience coming out of anesthesia, and as it wears off?

That depends on the type and depth of anesthesia you had. It also depends on the length of your surgery. A patient waking up from a thirty-minute procedure is going to feel quite a bit different than someone waking up after an eight-hour case.

You can expect to have very little, if any, memory of the procedure and the act of waking up afterward. Some patients experience what we call *retrograde amnesia*, meaning they have no memory of a point prior to receiving anesthesia. Some don't even remember the day of surgery at all. For example, they may have anesthesia at noon, and after it wears off they don't even remember waking up that morning at six. That is completely normal. It does not mean they had a bad reaction to the anesthetic.

One's ability to metabolize the various medications and chemicals that are used during the procedure can affect how one feels afterward. Everyone is different. That said, you can expect to feel unsteady on your feet. You may have an upset stomach and nausea. If you have severe nausea and you are sick to your stomach, call your physician's office. There are medications to help with that.

You can also expect to feel groggy for a period of time after waking up. In fact, you may be pretty darn loopy for a while. Be careful! I once had a patient who had a procedure with anesthesia in the morning. She went home later that day and started browsing on eBay to pass the time. A couple of weeks later, yellow sweaters started arriving in the mail. She had no idea why. She checked the purchase orders for all the shipments and sure enough, she discovered that all those yellow sweaters had been ordered on the evening of her procedure. She had zero memory of making those purchases. And she didn't even like yellow! I couldn't stop laughing. She offered me a free yellow sweater.

So take my advice: stay off the Internet and make no important decisions, purchases or phone calls until you are absolutely certain that you are "all there."

Immediate Post-Op

Make the most of yourself, for that is all there is of you.

Ralph Waldo Emerson

Question 36: Am I going to feel a lot of pain when I wake up?

First of all, that depends upon the individual. Some people have a very high pain tolerance and feel little discomfort at all, but another patient would describe it as the worst pain of their life. Those are obviously two ends of the pain scale spectrum, but the truth is that pain really comes down to the individual experiencing it. That does not mean one is better or worse than the other. It just means that each person's physiology and nerve endings are set up in their own unique way. Some people simply feel it more than others.

Women usually do much better with pain than men. Even the average six-year-old girl will do much better than the average six-year-old boy in an emergency room situation or following surgery. If you are a man reading this, you might be scoffing at that statement because we guys are supposed to be tough and women are supposed to be the "weaker sex." But ask any surgeon and they will agree: women are built to withstand discomfort. That probably comes from having to put up with us men all the time.

The second thing that influences the amount of pain you feel is the type of surgery you have had. Surgeries involving bone and muscle are going to hurt more than a mole removal. In other words, the more invasive or aggressive the procedure, the more pain you can anticipate. You should expect that – it's normal. You can't have surgery and believe you won't have some discomfort afterward. As a child, you can't get bumped in the nose by your brother and not have some pain. As an adult, you can't get bumped in the nose by a rhinoplasty surgeon and not feel some soreness.

As for managing that pain: some people do perfectly fine with Tylenol or Ibuprofen, and other people require a hefty dosage of controlled drugs to deal with their pain. It is always better to minimize the use of controlled drugs because they have side effects ranging from nausea to sedation to constipation to upset stomach, etc. Controlled drugs are controlled for a reason. You can ask Whitney Houston and Heath Ledger about that. Well, on second thought, you **can't** ask them… and that's my point.

Controlled drugs are not to be taken lightly. If you don't need them, do not use them.

If you are a bit uncomfortable after surgery but are feeling generally okay, then that means that for the most part, you're fine. Just go with it. You will heal better if you just let it run its course. Your body understands what is going on and what it needs to do to recover. Without heavy-duty drugs, you can react to things better. You can live your life sooner and on a more efficient basis. How you manage your postoperative pain is an individual decision that's best left to you and your surgeon. But in my experience, the less controlled drugs a patient takes, the better the patient does.

At any rate, keep in mind that you have just been exposed to a lot of chemicals and anesthetic. Any pain medicines you ingest very early after surgery are probably going to have a heightened effect. Put another way, if you had a long general anesthetic, be very judicious and careful about your use of narcotic pain medicine shortly thereafter, because if you are already groggy and you are taking additional narcotic pain medicine with the idea of "staying ahead of the pain," you can end up overdosed. Pain medicine is only to be used if you need it, not as a preventative measure. Never take it in anticipation of pain.

Question 37: How will I know if my level of pain and rate of recovery are normal?

Before your surgery, you will likely receive a packet of preoperative information that includes, among other things, what most patients say it feels like after your particular surgery. Study that, and call your doctor if you have any questions.

Generally speaking, if you have slow progression over time to an achiness that comes and goes and that is controlled by pain medicines, then that is a normal postoperative course for pain management. However, if you experience something drastically different from what is described in your preoperative information, then that is a red flag. If you have horrible pain or swelling that is immediate in its onset, then something is wrong. It is probably worth a call to your surgeon's office.

Question 38: What should I expect for healing time, and when will I be able to return to work?

Again, this depends on the patient and the kind of surgery they had. Some patients simply heal faster than others, and in general, the more invasive the surgery, the longer the healing time. Patience is a virtue when it comes to healing.

As for returning to work, you have to take into account where on the body the surgery took place. Breast augmentation and abdominal surgery are quite painful, but they can be hidden underneath shirts and sports bras and no one will ever know. Nose and eyelid surgery are a different story. While you may be cleared to resume reasonable activity after a few days, you are still going to look like a car accident victim for a couple of weeks afterward.

Refer to the information in your preoperative packet. If the surgeon makes a particular recommendation there, it is because they believe it will lead to the best outcome for you. Follow your doctor's orders. Have reasonable expectations. I have had patients expect to go golfing the day after surgery, and they wonder why I forbid it. They just had surgery, for heaven's sake! It is surgery whether you have your knee reconstructed or your gall bladder taken out or your nose fixed. No one would have his or her knee reconstructed and three days later be wondering why he or she couldn't run on it.

Way back in the early days of my surgical training, we would have a steady stream of patients come in for appendectomies, which is a limited surgery usually done by an intern with attending staff supervision. The families would hold a vigil, waiting to hear whether or not their loved one pulled through. Yet today when I do a combination face lift, brow lift, blepharoplasty and liposuction case for five hours under a general anesthetic, the patient's husband will drop her off and say, "Here's my number. Call me when she's done."

It never ceases to amaze me when people view one surgery as serious and another as trivial. I think it's because cosmetic surgery has been glamorized to a certain extent. Appendectomies don't make the covers of *Glamour* or *Cosmo*; plastic surgeries do. The public just doesn't take it seriously. They should. It is surgery, and it takes time to heal.

Question 39: Will I need a driver and someone to stay with me? For how long?

If you have any sort of sedation – whether it's mild sedation with oral medication or general anesthetic – then you will absolutely need assistance afterward. Sedation affects your brain. If it is enough to make you unconscious, it is enough to alter your thought processes until all that medication wears off. So for the first 24-hours, you should not make any important decisions. Don't call your banker and commit to a new business venture ten hours after surgery. Also, you should not drive or operate machinery for the first 24-hours. I always tell my patients that if they are planning on driving home after surgery, at least allow me enough time to get off the road first.

The best way to ensure that you don't do anything foolish (like ordering all the yellow sweaters on eBay) or dangerous (like overdosing yourself) is to have someone by your side for the first 12- to 24-hours after surgery. When you are sedated, it is almost impossible to protect yourself. If you are tipsy and you trip over a towel on the floor, who will be there to help you?

Still, don't count on your mate to stand at your bedside and cater to your every need. Even the most loving mate may get weak in the knees at the thought of changing a bandage. If you're having extensive surgery, consider hiring a nurse or assistant during the first several days after surgery. Make your arrangements well in advance of your procedure, and have a backup plan in case the first person cannot make it.

Surgery is serious business, so take it seriously. This is not the time to be a martyr and try to go it alone.

Question 40: What are some specific things I can do to make the early days of my recovery easier?

First, get your skin and body into the best possible condition prior to surgery. Your body is an amazing machine with the unique ability to heal itself, but it needs your help. From the moment you make the decision to have a procedure, start drinking plenty of water, eat well and get moderate amounts of exercise. Do not bask in the sun. Plan to purchase wrap-around sunglasses, a hat, a scarf and perhaps camouflage make-up to protect you from the sun and hide your bruising during your recovery.

Before you go in for surgery, assemble everything you will need by your bedside for when you return home. Most surgeons recommend elevating your head at least forty-five degrees during recovery, so have sufficient pillows and bolsters standing by. If your surgeon has recommended cold compresses to reduce swelling and bruising after surgery, have them ready. The same with homeopathic remedies such as Arnica or Bromelain to minimize inflammation and bruising… purchase those in advance.

Decide on your wardrobe prior to surgery. You will not want to pull anything over your head until you are completely healed, so plan on wearing zip-up or button-up loose fitting garments.

Purchase or prepare a selection of soft comfort foods to make meals easier in the early days of your recovery. If you are having skin resurfacing or jaw or facial bone surgery, buy a baby spoon and an adult sip cup. Have all your prescriptions filled and draw up a schedule for taking your pills.

Relaxation is one of the most important parts of a comfortable recovery. De-stress your life. Plan to give yourself the gift of time by arranging for someone to do your yard work and feed your pets for a while. You have decided to make an important investment in yourself. Protect that investment by planning ahead, and you will be richly rewarded for many years to come.

Question 41: Are there restrictions during recovery? What is a reasonable timeline for returning to normal activities?

With the majority of plastic surgeries – whether they were done on the head or the body – one can return to the normal activities of daily living after a week or two. Clearance to do heavy lifting and strenuous exercise varies by the procedure. For facial procedures, we usually recommend people wait two weeks. For abdominal procedures and breast surgeries, it is typically up to six weeks.

Of course, all of this can vary depending on the patient's rate of healing. Some people heal faster and they are able to get back to activity sooner. Others take a bit longer. I always urge people to err on the side of caution. Don't rush it, but don't languish on the sofa, either. Lying in bed for a week would make anyone feel rotten, surgery or no surgery. Patients who are more active after surgery use less pain medicine and have fewer complications. So get up and move around just as soon as you feel able. This will help expand your lungs, improve circulation and prevent blood clots. Energy begets energy. Get moving and you'll feel better.

Question 42: How soon will I see the surgeon again after my surgery?

This varies from practice to practice. There are some practices where you don't see the surgeon at all afterward. For instance, I have taken care of patients of celebrity doctors and those patients were not allowed to ever see their surgeon again. They were cared for by nurses and physicians' assistants from then on. That was the agreement they made at the time of surgery.

In my practice, I see the patient the very next day, with follow-up visits at one week, one month and three months. Obviously, that timeline is modified if there are complications or other variations in the surgery. It depends on the patient's comfort level during the recovery period, too.

Always remember that you are the customer, and you deserve great customer service. However, expecting a surgeon to hold your hand every day for weeks after the procedure is beyond reasonable. If you want to call the surgeon two dozen times in the first four days after surgery, that is probably not going to be appreciated. And believe me, I have had that happen. One patient called me 26 times in seven days (21 in the first 72 hours!) with questions, concerns, and pleas for reassurance. Now, that is obviously way beyond normal. My office had provided her with excellent preoperative information that answered all of the questions she called about. Still, in her mind, her questions were appropriate. She was scared. She could not mentally process what was going on. She was having difficulty absorbing information. She was insecure. I couldn't fault her for that. There was no malice in her making all those calls; she was not trying to make my life miserable (even though she did). She was not doing that on purpose. It is natural to be scared afterward; to be anxious.

But that is why the preoperative information is so important. It is given to you for a reason – to provide you with the answers to your questions long before you have to ask them. And that is also why the support staff is so important. You will rely on them greatly after your surgery. Meeting them in advance and expressing your appreciation for their help is critical – especially in practices in which you won't have access to the surgeon following your procedure. These folks provide exemplary care and support, and they deserve our most heartfelt gratitude.

Question 43: Do people ever regret their decision in the early healing stages?

Yes, they do. In fact, studies have shown that one in three patients will even qualify as clinically depressed soon after surgery. Why? Because of a tricky little psychological state called *cognitive dissonance.* Cognitive dissonance occurs when a person holds two or more conflicting beliefs, values, opinions or ideas in their mind at the same time. This clash of competing thoughts can bring about mental, emotional and even physical discomfort.

Here's how it works with cosmetic surgery: in the weeks leading up to the procedure, the patient becomes super excited about how much better they are going to look after surgery. They believe with all their heart that they are going to look great. They even daydream about it. But in the surgery's immediate aftermath, the patient looks in the mirror and sees the exact opposite of their dream-come-true. They see their worst nightmare. They don't look great at all. In fact, they think they look terrible, and they are frightened.

This conflict between two beliefs ("I am going to look great!" versus "Oh good heavens! I look terrible!") is cognitive dissonance. It can wreak such havoc with your thought process that your brain calls for a shut down or a decrease in your body's serotonin and dopamine production. That makes you depressed, and can convince you that this is never going to turn out okay.

But the good news is that these feelings are normal. It is natural to be a bit anxious. I even explain in the preoperative information packet that being clinically depressed afterward is part of a patient's normal emotional defense mechanism. It is true with any big decision. Doubting the wisdom of your choice after plastic surgery is like having buyer's remorse after purchasing a car. You buy a Chevy and then two weeks later you see the car ads and think, "Drat! I should have bought the Hyundai. It was a better deal." And you beat yourself up.

Now that you have read about the likelihood of depression, if conflicting thoughts start messing with your head after your surgery, you will have enough insight to tell yourself, "This is what Dr. Koch talked about. This too shall pass." Those feelings will rise and fall much like the inflammation from the surgery. Inflammation comes and then it goes. Your anxiety will come and go as well. Expect it. Remember that it is normal. However, do talk to your surgeon if your depression lasts longer than a couple of weeks.

Question 44: Will I require post-op garments or supplies? If so, when and where do I get those?

In facial surgeries, you will probably have a postoperative dressing or wrap afterward. Some surgeons recommend a chin support and neck support for a few days following the surgery. You can always expect a splint on your nose after rhinoplasty, and bandages over any wound. In breast surgery, abdominal surgery and the like, compressive garments are the norm, even up to six weeks post-surgery.

In the vast majority of cases, these garments and supplies are provided by your surgeon's practice. They will put them on while you are still snoozing from the surgery. That way, you won't have to deal with the garments in your initial discomfort.

Question 45: Are you available to me in the evenings or on weekends if I have concerns?

The law says that someone *must* be available. Doing surgery and not being accessible afterward – either personally or through a qualified representative – is called *itinerant medicine*, and it is illegal. I cannot do a surgery in Miami and then fly to Chicago without making arrangements to have someone available to answer questions or otherwise care for my patient in my absence. That person may be a physician colleague, physician's assistant or a nurse. The important thing is that they are able to answer your questions and at least contact someone who can help you should you have a problem after surgery. This is not only the law – it is also a requirement of accreditation, being granted hospital privileges, and getting a medical license.

Before surgery, ask which phone number you should use if you have questions. Ask for the job title of the person you can expect to talk to when you make that call. None of those options – nurse, PA, covering physician, etc. – is any worse or better than the next. It's just that knowing ahead of time will ease your mind and reassure you that if a problem does arise, you will know who you're dealing with.

Extended Post-Op

Plastic surgeons are always making mountains out of molehills.
Dolly Parton

Question 46: How long can I continue follow-up with my surgeon and/or support staff?

One to three months is the standard window for follow-up visits, depending upon the surgery. Some follow-up periods run from six months to a year. The normal healing process is usually complete by twelve months after surgery, so rarely does it extend beyond that.

However, I always tell my patients that they are stuck with me until they are happy with their results. That always makes them smile, but I mean it. As a surgeon, I have a secondary gain in my patients getting a great outcome. Word of mouth is powerful stuff. When one of my patients tells her girlfriends about what she had done and expresses her opinion of my skills and service, I want what she says to be positive. So within reason, my door is open for follow-ups until she is completely satisfied. I predict your surgeon will feel the same way.

Question 47: How long can I expect the results to last? How can I help maintain them?

This question has a two-part answer. The effects of the surgery itself are permanent. The skin we lift up and trim away at the time of a face lift is never coming back. So the best way I know to describe it is this: if a woman is 55-years old and we make her look 45 after surgery, when she is 65-years old she is going to look 55. She will always have the benefits of having the surgery done, but we cannot stop the conveyor belt of time.

Now, if that patient continues to try and move backward on the conveyor belt, she will start looking unusual. She can't be 60-years old and try to look like she is 25. It would look ridiculous. However, I know 60-year olds who appear to be 40, and they look fantastic. The surgery has a lot to do with that, but so does the individual patient.

Maintaining your results is important. If you have your skin resurfaced and you choose to spend six hours in the sun every day afterward, expect to see the effects of six hours in the sun every day whether you have had surgery or not. If you want to go back to smoking or to eating horrible food and never exercising, you can expect results commensurate with that. But if you maintain a healthy, lean body through exercise and proper nutrition, you will always benefit and your results will last longer. You will always be younger than your numerical age inside and out. That is true whether you've had surgery or not.

Remember, I am a doctor first and foremost. I always tell people that the first step toward looking great is to get healthy, get lean and detoxify. Whatever you do after that is icing on the cake. Just don't eat too much of the cake.

Question 48: Will weight loss or weight gain affect my results?

Yes, especially with body contouring procedures like liposuction. Here's why: you have a set number of fat cells in your body. When you gain weight, you don't gain more fat cells; the cells you already have simply get bigger. When you lose weight, those fat cells get smaller. When you have liposuction or liposculpture, we take some of those fat cells out. Since fat cells do not replace themselves, when we take them out they are gone forever. An aggressively liposuctioned area will not fill back up with fat afterward, even if you gain fifty pounds.

This is why it is not a great idea for an 18-year old to have liposuction. Eventually, that 18-year old is going to become a mature woman who gets pregnant and gains thirty pounds as a result. She will not gain weight in the areas that were liposuctioned, but she WILL gain weight in all the areas that weren't. That is going to look a bit unusual. It's like a young guy getting a hair transplant to cover up a bald spot in the front of the hairline. Those transplanted hairs are there forever. But the rest of his hair? Not so much. One day he'll be a 50-year old man with a Greek ring of hair around the side of his head, and a little tuft right in front where the hair transplant was done. Again, that's going to look a bit unusual.

So you have to understand that the processes of life and the changes that occur with time are going to continue. They will not stop just because you have had a surgery. You must maintain your results by staying healthy and lean. And if you are very young, make your decisions judiciously.

Question 49: What are my options if I am not happy with the results?

This is one of those questions you definitely need to know the answer to before crossing the cosmetic surgery bridge. It is essential that you ask this question up front, and also do your due diligence ahead of time. In other words, this is where the preoperative photos come in. This is where getting lots of opinions from reliable sources comes in. This is where talking to other patients comes in. This is where the preoperative meeting of the minds between you, your surgeon, and the support team comes in.

In the unlikely situation that you are unhappy with your results, open communication with your doctor and staff will be critical. Maintaining rapport with them is always important, no matter how frustrated you may be. It is essential for you to remember that firing hurtful barbs and being malicious to your surgeon will not inspire kindness in return. I know a few surgeons who need to learn that as well. While it is crucial for you to be calm and respectful, the doctor also has a responsibility to be calm and respectful and to uphold their commitment to a good outcome. If a surgeon is a jerk to you, she is not helping the situation. Studies prove that patients do not sue doctors they like personally. Doctors who are jerks are the ones who get sued.

So if you have a problem or a concern – such as an incision or contour changing shape, or looking worse rather than better – absolutely let your doctor know. He doesn't want a less than ideal outcome either. He wants you to tell your friends what a great surgeon he is.

BONUS QUESTION: Is plastic surgery addictive? Why do some people seem to not know when to stop?

According to the American Society of Plastic Surgeons (ASPS), there are two types of patients who undergo plastic surgery. There are patients who possess a strong self-image and would like to have a specific physical characteristic improved or changed, and there are those who have a physical defect or cosmetic flaw that has diminished their self-esteem over time. You should have plastic surgery for the right reasons. That's why this book is so important. If it is a **constant** search for self-esteem driving the desire for plastic surgery, the problem may extend beyond the doctor's office. By that I mean that the problem may be above the ears, so to speak. Some people are never satisfied, no matter what they have done. They want more – a "touch-up" or "just a little tweak."

Everything in moderation – and that applies to plastic surgery, also.

Body dysmorphic disorder (BDD) is defined by DSM-IV-TR (the diagnostic and statistical manual of psychiatry) as a condition marked by excessive pre-occupation with an imaginary or minor defect in a facial feature or localized part of the body. Often, patients with BDD will continue to seek more and more surgery to remedy a minor or imagined deformity. Sound like anyone's nose we know? Yep. Does everyone who has had a lot of plastic surgery have BDD? Certainly not. As mentioned earlier, good surgeons know when not to operate. Patients need sound opinions and smart recommendations before considering plastic surgery at all, whether it's their first, or another of many. As an old saying goes, "Sometimes the gap between 'more' and 'enough' never closes."

If you've read this far in this book, you are a smart consumer and you are making informed decisions. I trust you will choose a great surgeon should you decide to proceed with surgery. Just because you want to look great and improve a part of you doesn't mean you are on a slippery slope. Just travel safely.

And don't order any yellow sweaters. (

QUESTIONS TO ASK
YOURSELF

Motivations

She got her looks from her father. He's a plastic surgeon.

Groucho Marx

Question 50: Do I really need this? What is my primary motivation? What are my secondary motivations?

To have the best surgical outcome, it is important to understand your motivations. Having cosmetic surgery is a major decision. You are going to invest a lot of money and a lot of time in this. You are going to put your well-being at stake. You are going to trust another person to alter your appearance forever. In the vast majority of cases, that decision results in a delighted patient.

Still, you must ask yourself, "Why do I want to do this?" "I" is the key word in that sentence. You, the patient, have to want it. Not your husband who wishes you had bigger boobs. Not your modeling agent who wants you to have a smaller nose. Not your friends who all had cosmetic surgery and think you should too, because it will make them

feel better about their decision. Other people's hopes and dreams and rationales are **never** good reasons for you to have cosmetic surgery. Neither is having a procedure with the hope that someone who left you will come back. That is nothing but a fantasy.

No, you have to make this decision for you and you alone. Make this decision in a vacuum. If it is the right decision for you, it will be an obvious one. If it is not so obvious, then think of the secondary pros and cons. What are the cons? Well, there is some recovery time. There are some incision lines. There is some discomfort. There is an expense. And what are the pros? Feeling great about yourself for the rest of your life. Loving the way you look in the mirror. Loving how your clothes fit. Wearing a bikini with the same size top and bottom. Those are all wonderful benefits. In most cases, they far outweigh the drawbacks.

Take some time to think about your pro and con list. Actually write it all down and refer to the list often. Discuss it with the surgeon. Be honest with your doctor and yourself.

Question 51: Am I honestly prepared to follow my surgeon's orders and make all the lifestyle and habit changes he/she recommends before and after surgery?
This isn't just about having the surgery; it is about making a change for the better. If you are truly motivated to make

yourself better through cosmetic surgery, then you should also care enough about yourself to eat a healthy diet and get plenty of exercise. You should also care enough to quit smoking, and to cease using drugs and drinking alcohol to excess.

Listen, we all have our vices. I do. I am not going to stand on a pedestal and demand that you be perfect before you can be perfect. None of us are and none of us will ever be. But if you truly want your very best outcome with the plastic surgery, changing these other things along the way will make the road so much smoother. These vices are obstacles between you and your best result. If you have liposuction yet you are going to continue to gain weight, you are just setting up a roadblock for yourself. Trust me, that is a road you are going to have difficulty traveling. You are not going to be happy with your outcome. If you are not going to be happy with your outcome and you know it, why spend the money?

If you are married, you are not alone in investing that money. It is your spouse investing that money in you as well, to make you happy and to help you feel better about yourself. If you can't make positive changes for yourself, then at least do it for the person who is contributing financially and emotionally to your result – your spouse or your significant other. You are spending someone else's money on this too, so perhaps you ought to spend it wisely and do the right thing. How would you feel if you wrote a hefty check for their surgery and then they didn't follow through with any of the recommendations or take the appropriate precautions? They are essentially wasting money on an outcome they are going to be frustrated with. You would not want that, so don't behave that way yourself.

Either go all in, or don't go at all.

Expectations

You yourself, as much as anybody in the entire universe, deserve your love and affection.

Buddha

Question 52: What are my expectations? How will I deal with an outcome that doesn't match them?

Reasonable expectations are the foundation of cosmetic surgery. The ideal cosmetic surgery patient is a person who has a specific aspect of herself that she wants changed. She has thought about it for a long time and she has a reasonable expectation of the outcome. She has a logical understanding of the healing process. Let's go through those in detail.

If you don't know what you are seeking, then don't seek it. That would be like getting on a sailboat not knowing where you would like to go, and then not putting up a sail, either. That would be a foolish voyage. You are going nowhere, friend. Have a specific thing you want changed, and be able to articulate it clearly.

Think about it for a long time. Do your due diligence. Do a ton of research about what you are considering. This is a serious decision. Use your head.

Have a reasonable expectation of the outcome. There is a funny saying in this business that you can only climb so many rungs up the beauty ladder. Unless you are Cindy Crawford to start with, you are not going to look like Cindy Crawford afterward. If you start at the bottom of the ladder, you can expect to move up a rung or two, but not everyone has been dealt a royal flush in the card game of life. There are some things that simply cannot be changed. You must have reasonable expectations for what you can achieve, and those reasonable expectations can be attained through research, through your consultations with your surgeon and their staff, and through consultations with your family and your friends. They will help keep you grounded, because if you tell them you are going to look like Brad Pitt when your surgery is done, they will tell you that you are not. And that is a reasonable thing for them to say. There is no malice in that. They are saying it because they care about you, and because it's true.

You must have a logical understanding of the healing process. Again, I have people expect to have a facelift and eyelids done on Friday and then go back to work on Monday. I always wonder what in the world they are thinking. Pull your head out and understand that this is surgery. We are cutting into skin and moving it to a different place. You are going to bruise and swell and have inflammation. You are going to have discomfort. You are going to be frustrated early on with the healing process. It is going to take a minimum of a week or two to get back to looking even the slightest bit socially acceptable.

If your outcome is not what you expected and you are disappointed, it is quite likely that your surgeon is disappointed, too. Communicate! Be calm! Remember that you both want the same thing: a great outcome. There are tweaks, tucks and touch-ups done all the time in the plastic surgery business. There are remedies to make it better, to make things okay.

Except when there are not.

If a catastrophic complication has occurred, sometimes there is not a remedy for that. This is exceedingly rare, but as I mentioned earlier in this book, someone wins the lottery somewhere every week. Unfortunate things can and do happen. In those cases, it takes accepting who you are and what you have now, and moving forward with that.

More often than not, though, it is better than it was before. Not perfect – just better. "Perfection" and "flawlessness" are not reasonable expectations for cosmetic surgery. "Better" and "improved" are.

Question 53: How will this procedure affect my self-esteem?

The short answer is "for the better." Far and away, research studies show that more often than not, people feel more confident after a cosmetic surgery. They feel more proud of themselves and are more outgoing and assertive than they were prior to the procedure. Liking what you see in the mirror makes you feel better about yourself. And when you feel better about yourself, you exude positive energy, which is noticed by other people. And when people notice you for positive reasons, your life gets better.

There is an old saying that the most enthusiastic person in an argument always wins. When you are happy and enthusiastic, you do better all around. Studies show that even the act of holding a pencil in your teeth to create a smile makes you feel better inside. You feel happier after doing that. The point is that your body can change your mind. We often hear that our mind can change our body. Of course it can; we all know that we can make ourselves physically sick with stress and worry. But we can also make ourselves feel **better** by changing our body, whether it's through the way we position ourselves in a social situation, or the verbal and nonverbal language we use, or the eye contact we make – or by changing the shape of our nose, eyelids or breasts.

We all know that other people make judgments about us based upon our body language and our appearance. But did you know that we also make judgments about **ourselves** using those same criteria? Social psychologist Amy Cuddy of Harvard Business School studies nonverbal expressions of power and dominance. She and her colleagues found that people who were told to assume certain "power poses"[2] – such as standing tall with their hands on their hips, or sitting with their feet propped up on a table – for as little as two minutes experienced increased levels of the hormones that make human beings feel more confident. They also found that people who were told to assume "low power poses" – such as sitting or standing hunched over, with the arms close to the body – experienced a decrease in those same hormones affecting confidence.

The researchers then put both sets of people in pretend job interviews that were extremely stressful. And guess what? The "power pose" people performed much better than their "low power pose" cohorts. They appeared more confident, enthusiastic, and knowledgeable. In a nutshell, tiny tweaks in the way they positioned their bodies for just two minutes led to big changes in their internal chemistry, and consequently, their confidence levels and overall success.

2

http://www.people.hbs.edu/acuddy/in%20press,%20carney,%20cuddy,%20&%20yap,%20psych%20science.pdf, accessed October 11, 2012.

What does this mean for you? When you partner with a skilled, caring plastic surgeon to make a positive change in your body through cosmetic surgery, that change not only affects you on the outside. It affects you on the inside, too. You will feel more confident. You will be happier and more poised in every aspect of your life. I see this happen every day, and it never ceases to amaze and inspire me.

It is especially wonderful to see a young person blossom as a result of cosmetic surgery. Many years ago, I had an 18-year old patient who had huge, prominent ears. He had been teased relentlessly for his entire life. As a result, he was very quiet and always kept to himself. As soon as he turned 18, he told his mom that he wanted cosmetic surgery to fix his ears, and thankfully, she agreed to help him get it done. He told me in the consultation, "I am sick and tired of getting crap about my ears." We did an otoplasty to bring his ears back into an aesthetic anatomic position, and he was thrilled with the results. His personality changed completely. He came out of his shell. For the first time in his life, he was happy and comfortable in social situations. He never thought twice about his ears after that. He was like a new person, and all I did was change the shape of his ears.

Ten years later, I still get Christmas cards from his mother.

Impact on Everyday Life

You are here to enable the Divine Purpose of the Universe to unfold. That is how important you are.
Eckhart Tolle

Question 54: Are my friends and family supportive?

If the people who are the closest to you – the people you trust to help you make major life decisions – are not in any way supportive of your desire for plastic surgery, there might be a good reason. They might have your best interests at heart. They might actually be on your side. If, across the board, those people who love you tell you that you should not have cosmetic surgery, then you should listen. Ask yourself how might they benefit if you *don't* do it? Nothing will change for them if you choose not to. If they thought it would be great for you to do, they would probably encourage it.

I often meet with parents who are supportive of changing a hump on their teen daughter's nose. They say things like, "I think this will be great for her. She has given this a lot of thought, and she has wanted this for years. She's so beautiful inside and out, and this will just add to that." The patient and the parents are happy after the surgery, and it is exciting to see.

If a family member or friend is adamant that you should not have cosmetic surgery, ask yourself what their motivation might be. Maybe it has nothing to do with your best interests. Maybe a jealous boyfriend doesn't want you to change because if you felt better about yourself, you might leave him. I have seen that situation many times, too.

You have to consider everyone's opinions with a clear head. You want to have the backing of your family and friends. You are going to have to rely on them, in many cases, for your postoperative care and emotional support. But in the long term, these are people who will also have a big impact on your self-confidence going forward. You are a product of your environment, and your environment includes the people with whom you spend most of your time. They will definitely affect how you feel about your outcome.

I bet you have asked friends or family members for their opinions about which car you should purchase. Whether or not to have cosmetic surgery is the same thing. Ask them; see what they think. In most cases, they are going to be supportive of you. But if there is one outlying person who is not, then there may be ulterior motives. If everyone in your life is cheering you on but that jealous boyfriend is trying to block your path, then you may need to change more than just your nose. Just sayin'.

Question 55: What will I say if people ask if I have had plastic surgery?

This varies from one end of the spectrum to the other, but the pendulum has swung in the last ten years toward more open, honest communication about having plastic surgery. More people are willing to admit that they have had work done, and I love it. Why? Because it makes for happier people. When you tell others about what you've had done and you share your excitement, people will be excited along with you. If you try to hide it, you will feel bad and they will, too. A person who looks dramatically different yet claims to have never had plastic surgery... there is another name for that person, and it is "liar." That is not a good thing. You wouldn't buy a new car and then try to tell your neighbors that you didn't. They are looking right at the shiny red sports car in your driveway. Don't try to pretend you did not buy one.

If you are worried that the people in your office might gossip about your new-and-improved appearance, then the thing to do is to march in on your first day back after surgery and declare, "Hey guys! I've had my eyes done. I was SO tired of looking like a hound dog. What do you think? Do you like them?" Poof! The gossip is over before it began. There will be no talking behind your back because you have eliminated the need for it. You have been proactive.

So my advice is to be open and honest about the whole thing. Not having anything to hide is a great way to live your life. Be up front about who you are. Be confident in the results you have achieved, and move forward. Remember that what other people think of you is their business, not yours. Don't worry about it.

Question 56: Is the timing right with regard to family obligations, work and finances?

This all comes down to communication with the people who are your partners in this endeavor – your family, friends and employer. After your surgery, you are going to have to rely on them for help physically, emotionally, professionally and financially. They ought to have a say when it comes to the timing of your procedure.

Financially speaking, if you are not in a position to afford a luxury like plastic surgery, then do not spend the money. Depleting your son's college savings to pay for a butt lift is not in your child's best interest. If your mate is already working two jobs just to make ends meet and you want to have liposuction, you had better have his or her total buy in before you write that check. That said, making smart investments isn't limited only to buying real estate, stocks and bonds. You can make investments in yourself, too. But you have to consider all the other people who are affected by the cost of those investments. You have to do what is right for you and your family in the long run.

The impact of cosmetic surgery on a family is not only financial. If Mom is always gone having her breasts augmented and her lips plumped and is therefore not participating in her child's life, then that is bad. Mom may think she is pretty, but that does not make her a good mom. First priorities are "first" for a reason. Everything else has to take a back seat.

The same thing is true with your job. If you don't have vacation time to spare and you want to take two weeks off for elective cosmetic surgery, you are probably going to get in trouble. I have seen people try and pass off cosmetic surgery as medical leave. There is a fine line to walk there. Cosmetic surgery is a choice. Some companies allow medical leave for that, but most companies don't. Do not let having plastic surgery jeopardize your work life.

Family, work and finances... you have to take these things into consideration beforehand and make sure all the stars are in alignment before scheduling your surgery. Do the right thing. Otherwise, you will end up with worry and regret after your surgery, and that is the opposite of pretty.

Intuition

As soon as you trust yourself, you will know how to live.
Johann Wolfgang von Goethe

Question 57: Is the surgeon someone I feel comfortable with?

How you feel about a doctor is vitally important, even if you cannot explain exactly why you feel the way you do. We don't fully understand human intuition, or those "gut feelings," but I believe that if you have them, usually there is a good reason behind it. Where there's smoke, there's fire.

A 2002 study conducted at Harvard, the University of California-Riverside and the University of Toronto proved that point. A research team led by Nalini Ambady PhD studied film clips of surgeons' interactions with their patients, and scored the surgeons on how domineering or kind they were. What they discovered was fascinating. The researchers determined that "surgeons' tone of voice in routine visits is associated with malpractice claims history."[3] In other words, surgeons who were rated as domineering and uncaring in their communication with patients were also

---

[3] http://www.wjh.harvard.edu/~na/surgeons%20tone%20of%20voice.pdf, accessed October 10, 2012.

the surgeons who had been sued the most often for malpractice.

Put yet another way, doctors who are more likeable and empathetic in their conversations and dealings with their patients are far less likely to get sued than their more overbearing peers. And if a doctor has not been sued very often, it probably means that they had fewer complications and bad outcomes. Likeability and kindness play a big role in that.

If you think a surgeon is rude or seems like he doesn't have time for you, it is probably because that's the way he is. Move on. Choose someone you like. Choose someone you trust. You are putting your life in their hands. If you don't like that person, don't give them that gift, because they have not earned it.

Question 58: Did I feel a friendly connection with the staff? Did I feel at ease in the office?

As we discussed in an earlier question, the staff is going to play a giant role in your outcome, in your follow up visits and your phone calls. If you feel comfortable with them, they probably feel comfortable with you. And if they feel comfortable with you, they are going to be on board to help you.

It's like when you go to a restaurant. If you want to get great service, be nice to the waiter. The same is true at the surgeon's office. Establish a friendly rapport with the staff and they'll be more likely to engage in reciprocation for your kindness. If you want kindness, give it to them first. When you feel that kindness coming back to you, you can rest assured that they'll be on your side during your recovery period. Just as I mentioned earlier, if you are kind like Dorothy, you will get more help from the munchkins.

Question 59: Does the expected outcome outweigh the potential risks?

Asking yourself this question is foundational in any big decision you want to make. Whether you are purchasing stocks, investing in a marriage, or thinking about having cosmetic surgery, you have to ask yourself if it is worth the risk. You have to conduct a cost/benefit analysis. So whip out your pen and paper, make a list of pros and cons, and weigh the two sides against each other. Ask yourself and your support system – your family, your friends, your surgeon, the staff – *do you think this is really worth it?* Most of the time when a patient asks me that question, my answer is yes. But sometimes, my honest answer is no, I don't think so.

In that case, I am going to be a little standoffish. I will not recommend surgery for them. If they want to find someone who will do it regardless, they can, but it isn't going to be me. Then I remind them that this opinion is coming from someone who gets paid to do that surgery, yet I am still recommending they not do it. They know I am being honest with them. Sure, I would have a monetary gain from doing the surgery, but I would have a moral and reputational loss from doing it if the patient comes out unhappy with the outcome. So I am making a cost/benefit analysis as well. It has to be worth it to me to do that surgery, to feel that my patient is going to get a good result. I want to be able to sleep at night.

More often than not, my cosmetic surgery patients make sound decisions. More often than not, my patients are in the office for all the right reasons. More often than not, my patients have reasonable expectations, and they are confident that the value of the outcome will be worth more than what they have invested.

And more often than not, we both win.

Conclusion

You are always with yourself, so you might as well enjoy the company.
Diane Von Furstenberg

Well, here we are. We've made it to the end of our Q&A session. Obviously, there were far more than 50 questions, but it made for a better title, don't you think?

I believe we have covered all the bases. You have learned exactly which questions to ask yourself and potential surgeons about plastic surgery. You have been given the most responsible answers to those questions. You have learned about the latest research into how cosmetic surgery can enhance your life, and you have been given links to places you can go on the Internet to learn even more.

But while the questions and information in this book are designed to give you the tools to make an informed choice about who will be your surgeon if you decide to have a procedure, there is one important factor that you must remember as you travel this path: there is no such thing as the perfect plastic surgeon. If you find someone who answers every one of these questions flawlessly, call me. I'd like to meet her and shake her hand. As with most things in life, you will have to take the good along with the less-than-perfect when it comes to making this decision. You will have to assemble all the evidence and then take your time sifting through it with a logical mindset, and then pick the surgeon who feels right for you.

So I've given you the toolbox, but the bottom line is that as the patient, you have to take responsibility for participating in the outcome. The answers to these questions help, but the most important thing is going in with a positive attitude, trusting your instincts, and following your surgeon and support team's instructions. When things go well, celebrate with your surgeon. If things don't go so well, rely on your surgeon and support team to help you. Listen to what they have to say, because they want you to have a great outcome, too. Remember that the vast majority of complications work themselves out to a satisfactory result. They are usually nothing more than a bump in the road, and after a small detour, the patient makes it to their desired destination.

It makes my occupation better when patients have happy outcomes, even when I am not the one who does the surgery. It makes it easier for me to do what I love, which is helping people feel better about themselves. When patients like you are well-educated and making smart decisions, it makes everybody's outcome better. It means that I won't have to constantly have the Joan Rivers and the Michael Jackson nose conversations over and over and over... and over. If everybody had fantastic results, then people would be lining up to have plastic surgery all the time.

So even though I will probably never have the honor of knowing you, I honestly hope you get the results of your dreams. I sincerely hope that this book helps you along on your journey. I wish you a safe, happy and beautiful voyage, my friend!

Acknowledgments

To Pamela Suarez: You are the best! Thank you for your input, direction and literary expertise.

To Daphne Christensen: Thank you for being a team player, manager and coach all-in-one.

Thank you to my wife, Heidi: the most beautiful person I know; and my children: Nicole, Blake, Tatum and Piper. More than the stars and the moon.

About the Author

Brenton Koch, MD, FACS, is a board-certified facial plastic and reconstructive surgeon. He is certified by both the American Board of Facial Plastic and Reconstructive Surgery and the American Board of Otolaryngology - Head and Neck Surgery. At his practice in Des Moines, Iowa, plastic surgery of the face is his exclusive specialty. Dr. Koch is supported by administrative and operating room staffs that are specifically trained to care for plastic and reconstructive surgery patients. Each year this team of professionals prepares for and performs hundreds of facial surgeries treating conditions relating to appearance, accident, or disease.

Dr. Koch completed his undergraduate and pre-medical training at Drake University in Des Moines. He graduated from the University of Iowa College of Medicine, where he received numerous honors including the Hancher-Finkbine Medallion for outstanding academic leadership contributions to the University of Iowa College of Medicine. He also earned the American Medical Association National Leadership Achievement Award, which is presented to only twenty recipients nationally.

Dr. Koch completed residency at the prestigious University of Iowa Department of Otolaryngology - Head and Neck Surgery, which consistently ranks as one of the top programs in the country. He subsequently completed advanced fellowship training in facial plastic and reconstructive surgery at Indiana University and the Meridian Plastic Surgery Center in Indianapolis through the American Academy of Facial Plastic and Reconstructive Surgery. He served as clinical instructor of facial plastic surgery at Indiana University, and is currently a clinical instructor of facial plastic surgery with the University of Iowa Department of Otolaryngology - Head and Neck Surgery. He has continued to maintain active involvement in clinical research, with numerous publications, research awards and national presentations to his credit.

Dr. Koch and his wife, Heidi M. Koch MD, an age management and functional medicine physician, reside in Des Moines with their four children: Nicole, Blake, Tatum and Piper. Dr. Koch enjoys sports of all kinds, and as a former college football player, Ironman and competitive bodybuilder, he avidly enjoys exercise. His favorite activities, however, are those spent with his family.

Dr. Koch is the founder of a charitable non-profit for underprivileged student athletes called Empower to Play, an avid supporter of numerous charitable organizations in his community such as the Animal Rescue League of Iowa,

Juvenile Diabetes Research Foundation, Mercy Medical Center's Mammogram Assistance Fund and countless others through donations of his time and services.